AF614775

Disorders of Consciousness - A Review of Important Issues

Edited by Kamil Hakan Dogan

Published in London, United Kingdom

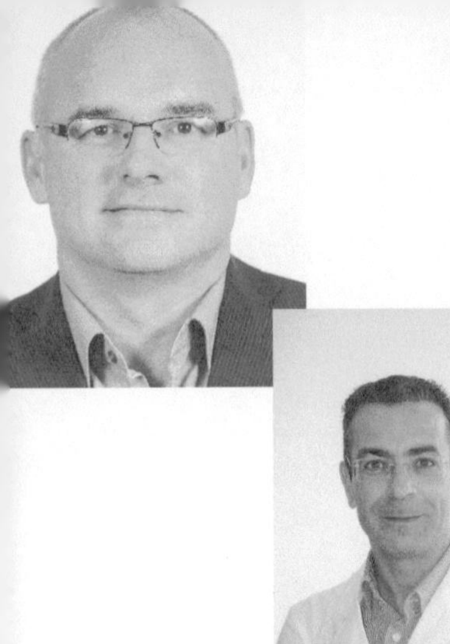
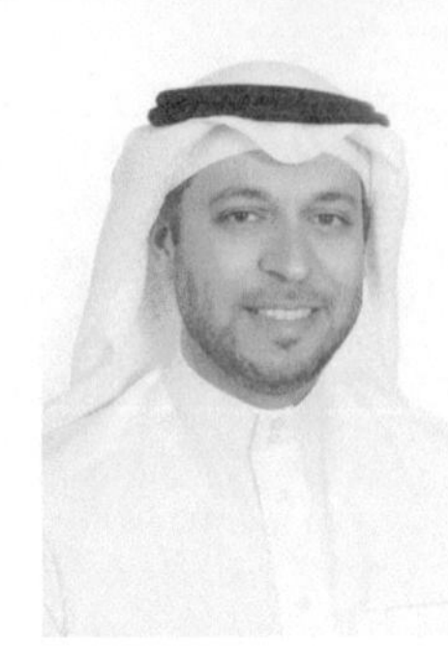
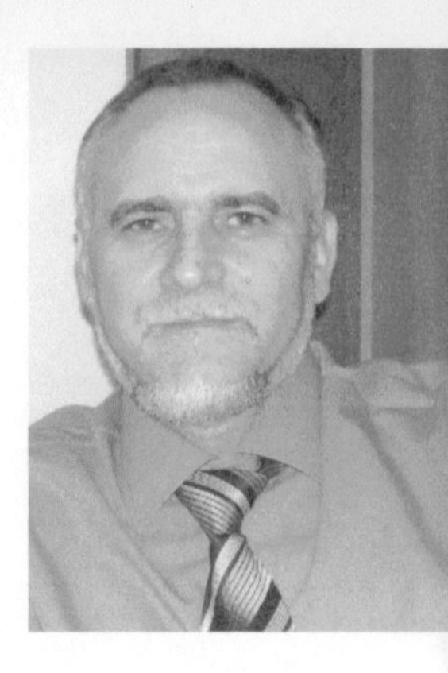
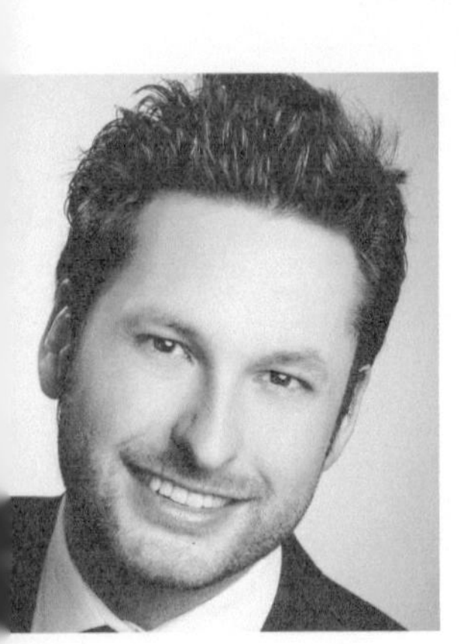
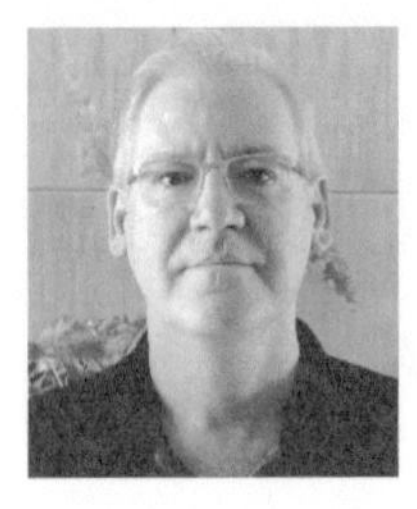
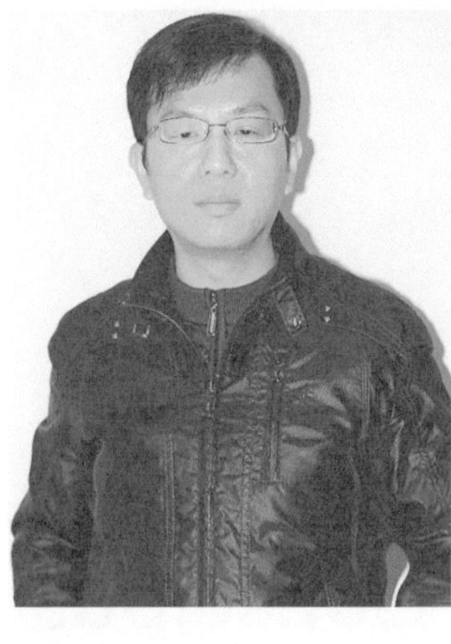

IntechOpen

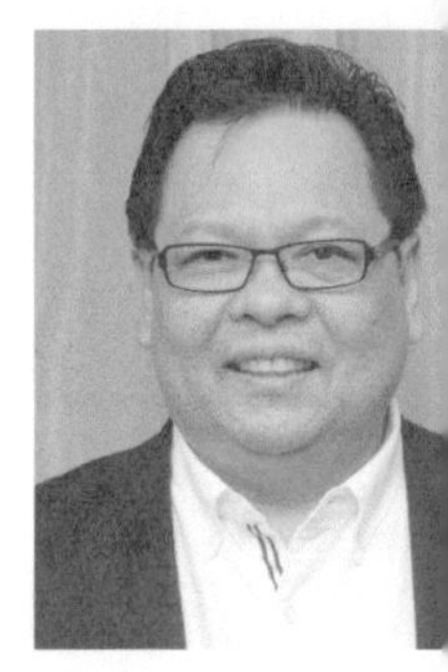
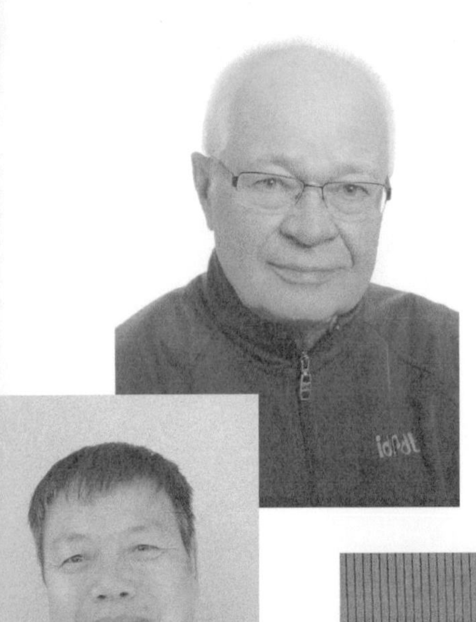
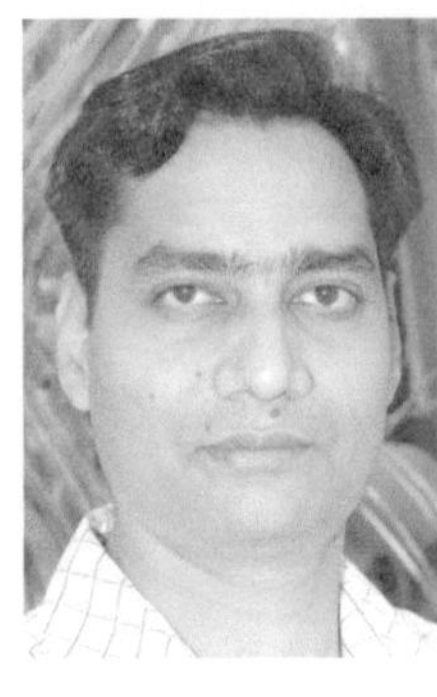
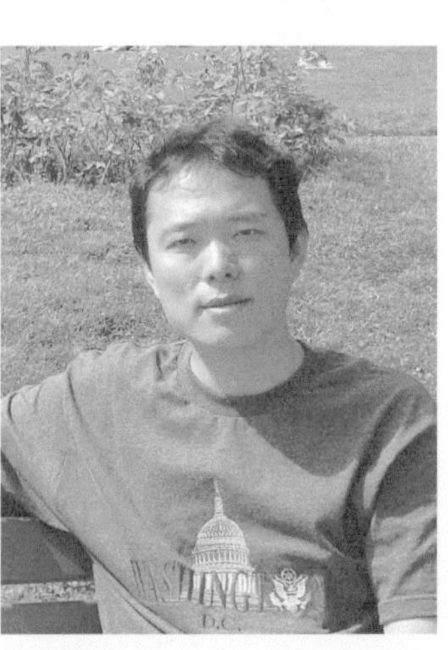
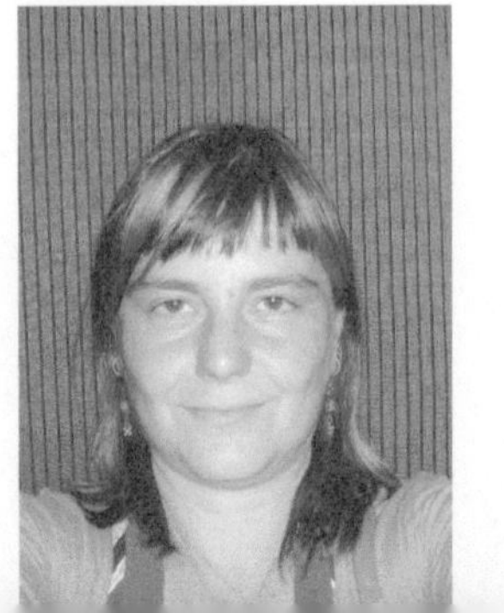

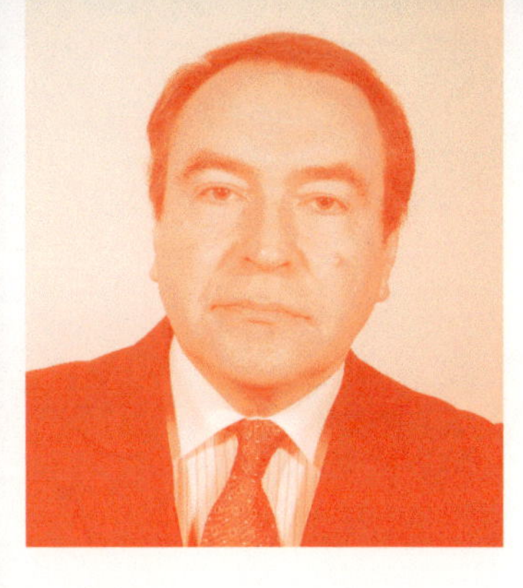

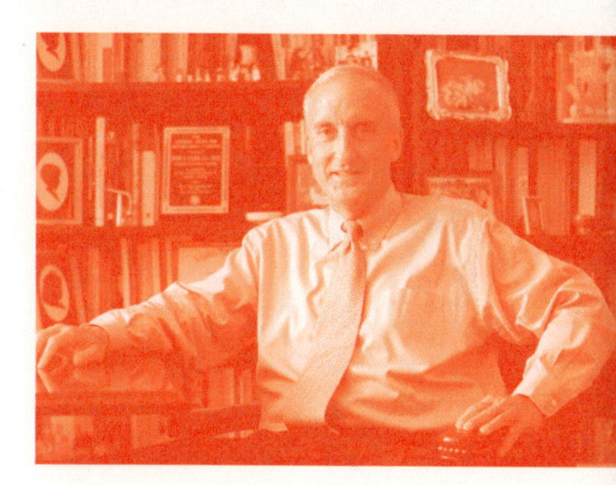

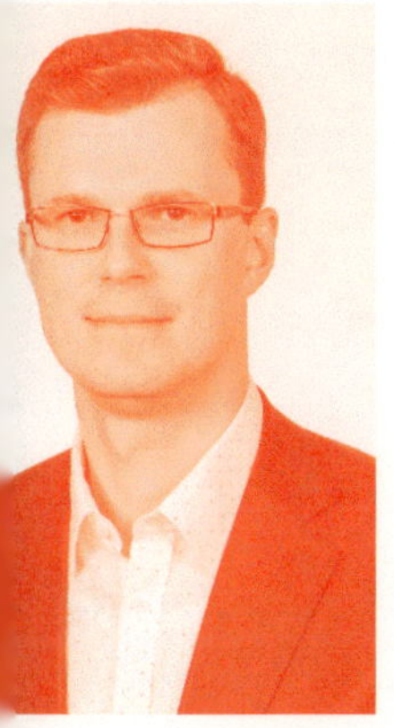

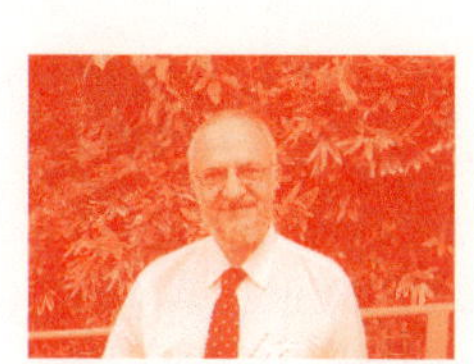

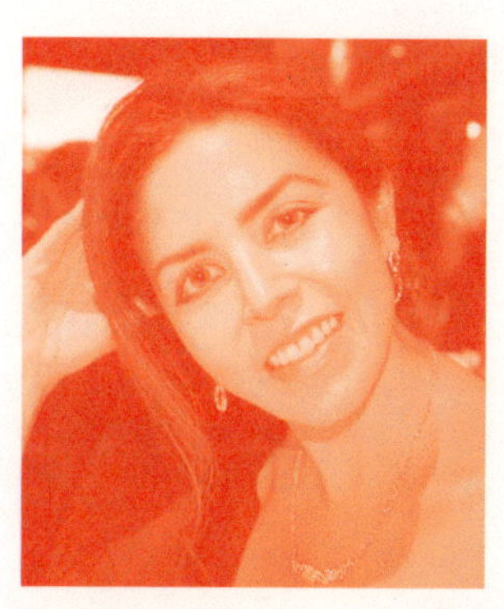

Supporting open minds since 2005

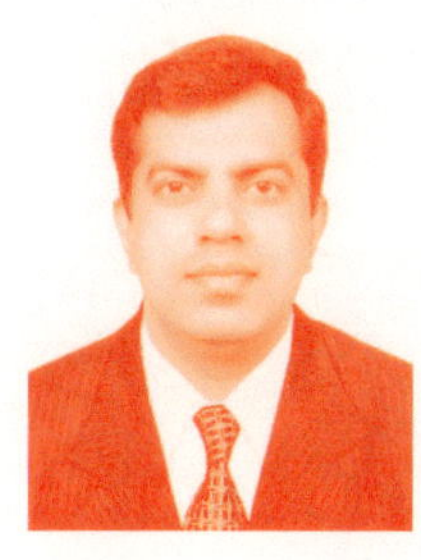

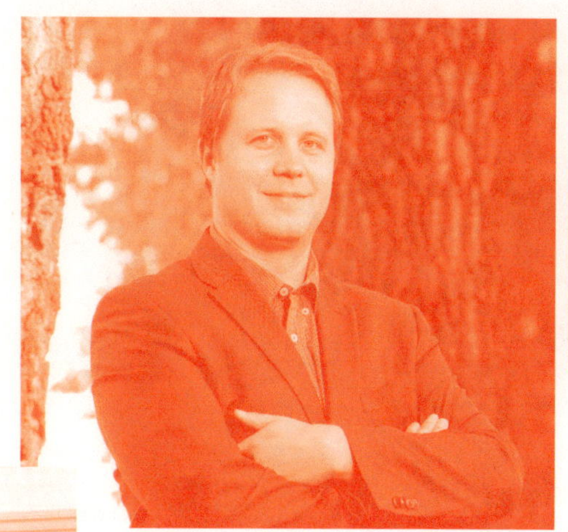

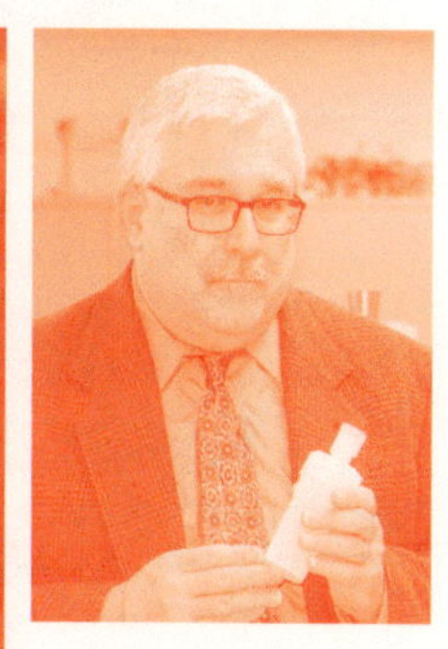

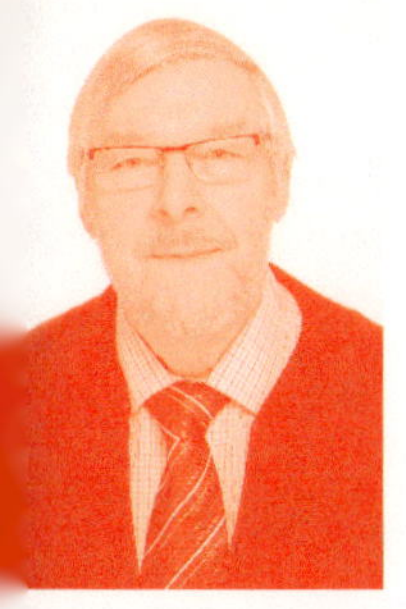

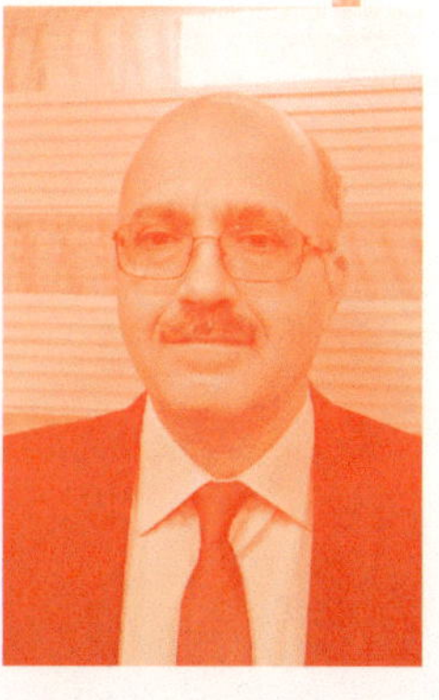

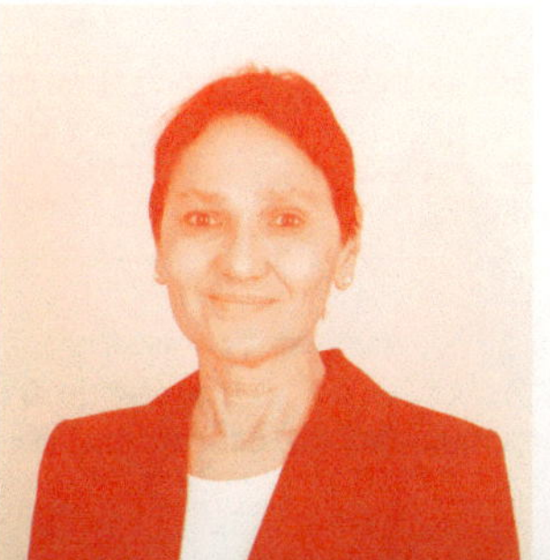

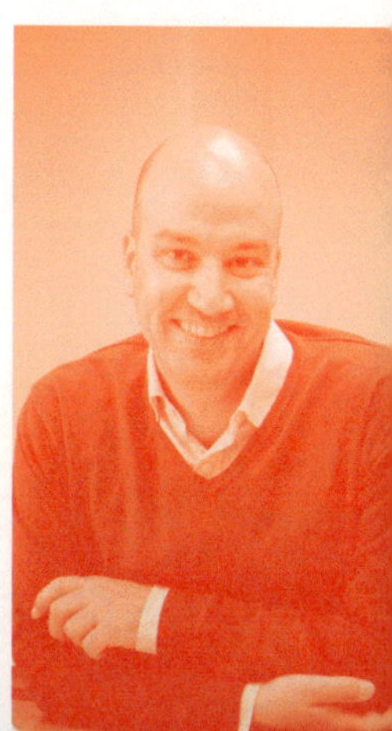

Disorders of Consciousness - A Review of Important Issues
http://dx.doi.org/10.5772/intechopen.78183
Edited by Kamil Hakan Dogan

Contributors
Urvashi Singh, Ashit Xess, Kiran Bala, Trond Flaegstad, Jai Jai Shiva Shankar, Sudharsana Rao Ande, Gülgün Uncu, Demet Ilhan, Oguz Erdinc, Demet Özbabalık Adapınar, Zeynep Özözen Ayas

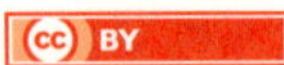

First published in London, United Kingdom, 2020 by IntechOpen
IntechOpen is the global imprint of INTECHOPEN LIMITED, registered in England and Wales, registration number: 11086078, 7th floor, 10 Lower Thames Street, London, EC3R 6AF, United Kingdom
Printed in Croatia

British Library Cataloguing-in-Publication Data
A catalogue record for this book is available from the British Library

Additional hard and PDF copies can be obtained from orders@intechopen.com

Disorders of Consciousness - A Review of Important Issues
Edited by Kamil Hakan Dogan
p. cm.
Print ISBN 978-1-78985-307-0
Online ISBN 978-1-78985-308-7
eBook (PDF) ISBN 978-1-78985-707-8

For EU product safety concerns:
IN TECH d.o.o., Prolaz Marije Krucifikse Kozulić 3, 51000 Rijeka, Croatia, info@intechopen.com or visit our website at intechopen.com.

Meet the editor

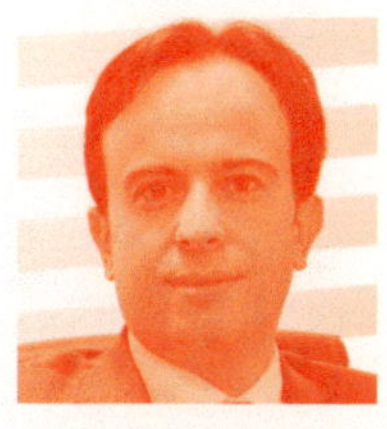

Kamil Hakan Dogan, MD, PhD, is a full professor and chair in the Department of Forensic Medicine at Selcuk University Faculty of Medicine in Turkey. Dr. Dogan received his MD from Gazi University Faculty of Medicine in 2000. After his extensive research in the field of forensic medicine, he received his PhD in Biochemistry in 2012. He gives lectures on forensic medicine and medical ethics to medical students as well as students of dentistry and law faculties. He is a reviewer in several international journals and has published over 200 articles in refereed journals, chapters in textbooks, and abstracts in scientific meetings. His publications have been cited more than 700 times.

Contents

Preface

Consciousness is a state of being awake and aware of one's self and surroundings according to the American Academy of Neurology. A conscious person is aware of things through thoughts and the five senses: sight, hearing, smell, taste, and touch. In disorders of consciousness, the patient has trouble being awake, or being aware, or both. There are advances in imaging techniques that contribute to the assessment of patients who have a disorder of consciousness. With neuroimaging techniques the information may be gathered about a patient's cognitive ability without having to rely on verbal or motor behavior. The prognosis of disorders of consciousness is highly variable. It depends on the cause, duration, and extent of the affected site. However, appropriate initial care and proper treatment are very important to prevent the occurrence of secondary damage and to accelerate patient recovery.

Thanks to advances in science and technology, we learn new information about diseases every day. This book includes current approaches to some important issues related to disorders of consciousness.

Kamil Hakan Dogan
Selcuk University Faculty of Medicine,
Department of Forensic Medicine,
Konya, Turkey

Chapter 1

Hypoxic Brain Injury

Zeynep Özözen Ayas, Gülgün Uncu and Demet Özbabalık Adapınar

Abstract

Hypoxic brain injury (HBI) is a clinical condition that results from a decrease in brain blood flow and oxygenation. The damage due to cerebral hypoperfusion is caused by many possible reasons, which leads to severe wide spectrum of clinical presentations. It can be difficult to manage disease process of HBI because the clinical outcomes are poor and treatment options are limited. Neuroprotective trials against different underlying pathophysiological pathways are promising. In spite of all the difficulties, promising signals are obtained in the recent studies. In this article, we aim to provide the details of neurotoxic mechanisms and new interventions for neuroprotection of HBI.

Keywords: hypoxic brain injury, neuronal death, treatment

1. Introduction

Hypoxic brain injury (HBI) is a clinical condition that results from a decrease in brain blood flow and oxygenation. Energy in the brain is mainly derived from oxygen and glucose by 95% oxidative metabolism [1, 2]. About 50% of the energy obtained is used for communication and synaptic activity between neurons, 25% for the passage of ions through the cell membrane and 25% for molecular transport and biosynthesis [3, 4]. Metabolic need increases in seizure and fever but decreases in deep coma and anaesthesia. HBI can be defined as a damage to brain cells due to hypoxia. In HBI, the clinical definition is more complex, indicating hypoxia with many etiologic causes, and broad-spectrum brain injury caused by ischemia with or without reperfusion. Clinic developmental stage of the brain, condition of development of damage, regional weakness, ethology, difficult predictability of treatment and outcomes are heterogeneous due to the differences in accepted guidelines and management standards. Although effective treatment has not yet been found, progress has been made in the prevention of HBI.

2. Hypoxic-ischemic brain injury

Encephalopathy—the neurologic syndrome composed of abnormalities of consciousness, tone and autonomic control is the hallmark of acute HBI [5]. The stage of encephalopathy depends on the timing and severity of the hypoxia. HBI is an important cause of mortality and morbidity in the paediatric age group. Although effective treatment has not been found yet, progress has been made in the prevention of HBI. Advances in conservation have been achieved with neonatal asphyxia

IntechOpen

and mild hypothermia in ventricular fibrillation after cardiac arrest in adulthood and early use of thrombolytics after embolic stroke in adults.

3. Cellular mechanisms of neuronal death following HBI

Neurons consistently require a source of metabolic substrates, especially glucose and oxygen. HI brain injury results from intracellular and intracellular processes during and after the imbalance of the presence and consumption of these substrates in the brain. In animal models, neuronal death after HBI occurs in two phases [6]: Immediately after HBI, neurons begin to die rapidly, possibly a cell death process characterised by necrosis, loss of acute plasma membrane integrity and loss of ATP [7]. In the second stage, neurons die from hours to days [8], primarily through apoptosis [9], which is cascade of active, tightly regulated intracellular pathways. Neuropathological evidence of classical neuronal apoptosis after HBI is less pronounced in humans than in animal models [10]. However, there is no doubt that urgent and delayed neuronal deaths are below neurological damage after HBI. New approaches to salvage neurons following HBI have strengthened the existing understanding of HI-induced brain injury mechanisms to specifically target central mechanisms of neuronal death. We will briefly review excitotoxicity, free radical toxicity and inflammation procedures in order to place these treatments in the context of their targeted cellular mechanisms.

3.1 Excitotoxicity

Glutamate is a stimulating neurotransmitter everywhere in the brain. Under pathological conditions, including HI, neuronal receptors for glutamate are overactive due to pathologically high glutamate concentration in the extraneuronal domain. This high concentration occurs as a result of synaptic release of glutamate pathologically, dysfunction of glutamate uptake mechanisms and release of glutamate from the intracellular metabolic pool. Glutamate receptor overactivation results in neuronal death, hence excitotoxicity. Overactivation of the N-methyl-D-aspartate (NMDA), subtype of the glutamate receptor, was highly effective in neuronal death after HI. NMDA receptor overactivation allows intracellular calcium to rise to toxic levels and causes cell death by activating cytotoxic phospholipases, proteases, lipases and endonucleases. Calcium is also absorbed by the mitochondria, causing loss of ATP synthesis, oxidative stress, release of proapoptotic factors and activation of the apoptotic cascade.

3.2 Free radical toxicity

Free radicals are molecules containing one or more unpaired electrons that allow increased intermolecular reactivity. Primary oxygen-free radical superoxide anion is produced in cells (O_2^-). Superoxide is an important intracellular signalling molecule, as is the metabolite hydrogen peroxide (H_2O_2). Together with the highly reactive hydroxyl radical, O_2^- and H_2O_2 are oxygen-derived free radicals present in the cell. Oxidative stress refers to increased levels of these radicals. Oxidative stress contributes to neuron death after HI [11], by breaking down cellular proteins and DNA.

In addition to oxidative stress, increased nitric oxide (NO), nitrogen-free radical, production is a central mechanism of HI-induced neuronal death [12]. Increased NO production is mediated by neuron-specific NO synthase (nNOS) and elevated by HI (and excitotoxicity)-induced intracellular calcium concentrations.

Endothelial NOS (eNOS), a second NO synthase isoform, controls vascular resistance in all organs, including the brain. Maintaining eNOS activity during and after experimental HI improves cerebral blood flow and neuronal survival [13]; therefore, treatments aimed at reducing neuronal NO production should specifically target nNOS and maintain eNOS activity. In addition to its direct effects, NO interacts with O_2^- to form highly reactive and toxic radical peroxynitrite [14]. Peroxynitrite-mediated peroxidation of lipid components of cellular membranes [15] and mitochondrial proteins oxidative modification [16] are important mechanisms of neuronal damage. In particular, lipid peroxidation changes the cellular membrane structure and function that triggers cellular necrosis or apoptosis.

3.3 Inflammation

Improved results in HBI animal models following inflammation inhibition [17] show that inflammation is an important mechanism of HI-induced neuronal death. After HBI, microglia is activated [18], proinflammatory cytokines, e.g. IL-1 and TNF-alpha. In addition, microglia-derived chemokines increase acutely to receive peripheral immune cells into the brain [19]. HBI activates the complementary stage in the brain [20]. Complement activation results in the formation of membrane attack complexes that form pores within the plasma membranes and lead to cell lysis [21]. Therefore, after HBI, a coordinated inflammatory response emerges, which makes a significant contribution to HBI-induced neuron death in the brain.

4. New treatments for HBI

The understanding of the mechanisms of HI-induced neuronal approaches to neuroprotection have shown promise in pre-clinical studies and early clinical trials. Below, we review some of the most promising approaches at different stages of development from early stage research to clinical studies and FDA approval. Since these therapies may address different mechanisms than those mediating hypothermized neuroprotection, these novel therapies also provide additional neuroprotection to those available from hypothermia therapy.

4.1 Erythropoietin

Erythropoietin (EPO) is an endogenous, hypoxia-derived glycoprotein produced in the kidney that has been shown to first regulate haematopoietic function through EPO-specific receptors. [22]. Recombinant EPO (r-EPO), currently approved to increase erythropoietin in anaemia, has also been shown in animal studies where HBI is neuroprotective [23, 24]. Activation of neuronal EPO receptors prevents HBI-induced activation of NMDA receptors and increases expression of anti-apoptotic proteins, potentially reduces excitotoxicity and reduces apoptosis [24, 25]. EPO receptor activation also inhibits HBI-induced stimulation of peroxynitrite (oxidative stress) and inflammatory cytokines, potentially reducing free radical toxicity and inflammation. [25]. EPO receptor expression, which is of particular importance for neonatal HBI, is abundant in the developing mammalian brain [26]. Systemically administered r-EPO after HBI has been shown to cross the blood-brain barrier [27]. In one study, the pharmacokinetics of EPO levels in cerebrospinal fluid in babies treated with EPO after HBI was parallel to that observed in serum [28], suggesting that r-EPO could cross the blood-brain barrier in humans.

4.2 Melatonin

Melatonin is a pineal gland hormone secreted in response to environmental light-dark cycles [29]. Melatonin has multiple cellular effects, two of which directly target known mechanisms of HBI. First, melatonin reduces free radical toxicity, scavenging hydroxyl radical and peroxynitrite by direct electron transfer [30]. Melatonin also reduces O_2^- production in brain slices in vitro following hypoxic ischemic stress [31]. Second, melatonin has anti-inflammatory activity. Thus, after umbilical cord occlusion in fatal sheep, melatonin reduced the production of 8-isoprostanes [32], a potent mediator of HBI-induced inflammation. In addition, melatonin given to rats immediately after focal cerebral ischemia decreased neutrophil migration and macrophage/activated microglial infiltration after 48 hours and decreased only in the ischemic hemisphere [33]. Finally, melatonin reduces the binding of NF-yaB to DNA, resulting in the production of proinflammatory cytokines including interleukin-2, interleukin-6 and tumour necrosis factor alpha [34]. These cellular effects have led to extensive investigation of melatonin as a treatment for hypoxic brain damage.

Short-term assessments of melatonin, infarct size and neurobehavioural outcomes in rats after focal cerebral ischemia are improved [33], suggesting that melatonin treatment may be applicable to global brain ischemia in the newborn. However, short-term improvements may reflect only the temporary inhibition of death-induced procedures without altering the final extent of neuronal death. Finally, melatonin may have a neuroproductive effect in addition to hypothermia. Following induction of global ischemia in newborn pigs, melatonin with hypothermia reduced MR spectroscopic indices of impaired cerebral energy metabolism compared to hypothermia alone [35].

4.3 Allopurinol

Allopurinol is a xanthine oxidase inhibitor that is a source of cytosolic O_2^-, which has attracted attention as a potential neuroprotective agent during HI, especially as it can cross the placenta to produce therapeutic levels in newborns [36]. Animal models including in vivo and in vitro rat models and in vivo sheep models have demonstrated that allopurinol is neuroprotective [37].

4.4 Topiramate

Topiramate is an anti-epileptic drug of interest as a potential neuroprotective agent for brain injury. Topiramate prevents seizures by inhibiting neuronal excitability, including blockade of glutamate receptors [38]. This potential anti-excitotoxicity effect suggests topiramate as a candidate treatment for HBI. Indeed, following carotid artery ligation in the rat, topiramate significantly reduces neuronal death through inhibition of glutamate receptor activity [39], reducing HBI-induced neuronal apoptosis [40]. Of particular interest is the observation that topiramate, when combined with hypothermia, adds neuroprotective effects in animal models. [41].

In the pilot study, topiramate associated with whole-body hypothermia in 27 asphyxia infants did not cause any adverse effects, short-term outcome differences or pathological cerebral magnetic resonance imaging incidence compared to 27 controls [42]. Further extensive clinical studies are needed to assess the efficacy of topiramate in preventing HI injury.

4.5 Xenon

Xenon is a chemically non-reactive gas that is extensively studied as a general anaesthesia in Europe [43, 44], due to its highly favourable safety profile. One of the activities of xenon is against NMDA receptor activation, which reduces excitotoxicity. This reduced activity results from the xenon glycine block that binds to its regulatory region on the receptor [45]. Following hypoxia or excitotoxicity in cultured murine neurons, increased xenon concentrations significantly increased neuronal survival [46]. In neonatal rats, xenon inhalation improved both histological and functional outcomes 2 months after global HI [47]. Similarly, following global forebrain ischemia in the newborn pig, xenon inhalation proved neuronal survival 72 hours after insult [48]. In particular, in these models, xenon-induced neuroprotection has been found to add to the neuroprotection provided by induced hypothermia.

4.6 nNOS inhibition

The central role of NO in HI-mediated neuronal injury and the presence of specific small molecule inhibitors of nNOS make nNOS inhibition a potentially attractive approach. With the discovery of the toxic role of NOS in HI, early studies of NOS inhibitors have yielded contradictory results since early inhibitors do not have isoform specificity [49]. However, newer, specific nNOS inhibitors may promise more [50]. Prophylactic use of highly specific nNOS inhibitor JI-10 in preterm fetal sheep increased neuronal survival following deep asphyxia [51]. Although initial data for selective nNOS inhibitors are promising, the extent of non-target effects, such as inhibition of eNOS activity and any accompanying reduction in cerebral blood flow, will need to be investigated to initiate clinical trials.

4.7 Pluronic co-polymers

After HBI, the functions of cellular membranes may change due to lipid peroxidation and lipid signalling changes. After severe HI, neuronal plasma membrane dysfunction leads to reduced membrane integrity, infiltration of intracellular components into the extracellular space and necrosis. When HI is not severe enough to induce necrosis, HI-mediated dysfunction of mitochondrial intracellular membranes can trigger apoptosis [52]. Recently, a class of synthetic molecules has been used to address HI-induced dysfunction of injured neuronal membranes in pluronic, in vitro and in vivo. Pluronics, which consist of poly [ethylene oxide] (PEO) and poly [propylene oxide] (PPO) chains, have been arranged in a three-block PEO-PPO-PEO structure. This structure allows the pluronics to interact with the cellular membranes [53, 54] and recovers the integrity of the plasma membrane after injury. Pluronic F-68, a member of Pluronics, has been shown to immediately rescue neurons from death in in vitro HI models by apoptosis blockage [55, 56]. Preliminary evidence also shows that Pluronic F-68, provided to animals for 1 week after HI, significantly improves neuronal survival in the hippocampus, a brain region highly sensitive to global HI, and saves hippocampus behaviour [57]. The novelty of this membrane-targeted approach and the lack of toxicity [58, 59] suggest that targeting membrane dysfunction may be a suitable treatment for future HBI.

4.8 Therapeutic hypothermia

The main mechanism underlying hypothermia in reducing ischemic tissue damage is its effect on metabolism [60]. Oxygen use decreases by 7% almost linearly with each °C reduction below normal [61]. On the other hand, ischemia becomes more tolerable due to the slowdown in metabolism, although a decrease in blood pressure of about 5% per degree has been observed. In animal experiments, the brain volume is approximately 4% less at 25°C compared to 37°C. Here, the main decreasing cerebral blood flow and volume, the CSF section increases by about 32%. In conclusion, intracranial and venous pressures decrease [62]. In addition, hypothermia reduces the release of excitatory neurotransmitters, such as glutamate and glycine, suppresses free radical toxicity, creates favourable effects on intracellular mediator systems, also reduces intracellular acidosis, inhibits the excretion of ubiquitin, which binds abnormal proteins and facilitates their excretion, anti-apoptotic effects and anti-inflammatory effects and other mechanisms by reducing ischemic neuron damage [63, 64].

5. Conclusion

Hypoxic-ischemic brain injury is a simple imbalance between demand and supply to brain energy. However, cellular mechanisms leading to neuronal death are complex and multifactorial. The overall effectiveness of induced hypothermia is relatively low and the need for mechanism-oriented therapies for HBI is high. Basic research may provide therapeutic targets for translation testing, while defining the underlying mechanisms of HBI-mediated neuronal death. The approaches discussed above target the cellular mechanisms of HBI-mediated neuronal death in many different ways. With ongoing research, one or more of these approaches or their derivatives may ultimately be effective treatments for HBI.

Author details

Zeynep Özözen Ayas*, Gülgün Uncu and Demet Özbabalık Adapınar
Department of Neurology, Eskişehir City Hospital, Eskişehir, Turkey

*Address all correspondence to: zozozen@hotmail.com

References

[1] Astrup J, Sorenson PM, Sorenson HR. Oxygen and glucose consumption is related to Na+, K+ transport in canine brain. Stroke. 1981;**12**:726-730

[2] Kassissia IG, Goresky CA, Rose CP, et al. Tracer oxygen distribution is barrier-limited in the cerebral microcirculation. Circulation Research. 1995;**77**:1202-1211

[3] Astrup J. Energy-requiring cell functions in the ischemic brain: Their critical supply and possible inhibition in the protective therapy. Journal of Neurosurgery. 1982;**56**:482-497

[4] Siesjo BK. Cerebral circulation and metabolism. Journal of Neurosurgery. 1984;**60**:883-908

[5] Sarnat HB, Sarnat MS. Neonatal encephalopathy following fetal distress. A clinical and electroencephalographic study. Archives of Neurology. 1976;**33**:696-705

[6] Northington FJ, Ferriero DM, Graham EM, et al. Early Neurodegeneration after hypoxia-ischemia in neonatal rat is necrosis while delayed neuronal death is apoptosis. Neurobiology of Disease. 2001;**8**:207-219

[7] Fricker M, Tolkovsky AM. Cell culture techniques. In: Acsher M, Sunol C, Bal-Price A, editors. Mechanisms of neuronal and glial cell death. NeuroMethods. New York: Humana Press; 2011

[8] McLean C, Ferriero D. Mechanisms of hypoxic—Ischemic injury in the term infant. Seminars in Perinatology. 2004;**28**:425-432

[9] Ankarcrona M, Dypbukt JM, Bonfoco E, et al. Glutamate-induced neuronal death: A succession of necrosis or apoptosis depending on mitochondrial function. Neuron. 1995;**15**:961-973

[10] Northington FJ, Chavez-Valdez R, Martin LJ. Neuronal cell death in neonatal hypoxia-ischemia. Annals of Neurology. 2011;**69**:743-758

[11] Abramov AY, Scorziello A, Duchen MR. Three distinct mechanisms generate oxygen free radicals in neurons and contribute to cell death during anoxia and Reoxygenation. The Journal of Neuroscience. 2007;**27**:1129-1138

[12] Moro MA, Cardenas A, Hurtado O, et al. Role of nitric oxide after brain ischaemia. Cell Calcium. 2004;**36**:265-275

[13] Huang Z, Huang PL, Ma J, et al. Enlarged infarcts in endothelial nitric oxide synthase knockout mice are attenuated by nitro-L-arginine. Journal of Cerebral Blood Flow and Metabolism. 1996;**16**:981-987

[14] Brown GC. Nitric oxide regulates mitochondrial respiration and cell functions by inhibiting cytochrome oxidase. FEBS Letters. 1995;**369**:136-139

[15] Szabo C. Multiple pathways of peroxynitrite cytotoxicity. Toxicology Letters. 2003;**140-141**:105-112

[16] Bolanos JP, Almeida A, Medina JM. Nitric oxide mediates brain mitochondrial damage during perinatal anoxia. Brain Research. 1998;**787**:117-122

[17] Liu XH, Kwon D, Schielke GP, et al. Mice deficient in interleukin-1 converting enzyme are resistant to neonatal hypoxic-ischemic brain damage. Journal of Cerebral Blood Flow and Metabolism. 1999;**19**:1099-1108

[18] McRae A, Gilland E, Bona E, et al. Microglia activation after neonatal

hypoxic-ischemia. Brain Research. Developmental Brain Research. 1995;**84**:245-252

[19] Bona E, Andersson AL, Blomgren K, et al. Chemokine and inflammatory cell response to hypoxia ischemia in immature rats. Pediatric Research. 1999;**45**:500-509

[20] Cowell RM, Plane JM, Silverstein FS. Complement activation contributes to hypoxic-ischemic brain injury in neonatal rats. The Journal of Neuroscience. 2003;**23**:9459-9468

[21] Harhausen D, Khojasteh U, Stahel PF, et al. Membrane attack complex inhibitor CD59a protects against focal cerebral ischemia in mice. Journal of Neuroinflammation. 2010;7:15

[22] Koury MJ, Bondurant MC. The mechanism of erythropoietin action. American Journal of Kidney Diseases. 1991;**18**:20-23

[23] Aydin A, Genc K, Akhisaroglu M, et al. Erythropoietin exerts neuroprotective effect in neonatal rat model of hypoxic-ischemic brain injury. Brain & Development. 2003;**25**:494-498

[24] Kumral A, Genc S, Ozer E, et al. Erythropoietin downregulates bax and DP5 proapoptotic gene expression in neonatal hypoxic-ischemic brain injury. Biology of the Neonate. 2006;**89**:205-210

[25] Digicaylioglu M, Lipton SA. Erythropoietin-mediated neuroprotection involves cross-talk between Jak2 and NF-kappaB signalling cascades. Nature. 2001;**412**:641-647

[26] Juul SE, Anderson DK, Li Y, et al. Erythropoietin and erythropoietin receptor in the developing human central nervous system. Pediatric Research. 1998;**43**:40-49

[27] Brines ML, Ghezzi P, Keenan S, et al. Erythropoietin crosses the blood-brain barrier to protect against experimental brain injury. Proceedings of the National Academy of Sciences of the United States of America. 2000;**97**:10526-10531

[28] Zhu C, Kang W, Xu F, et al. Erythropoietin improved neurologic outcomes in newborns with hypoxic ischemic encephalopathy. Pediatrics. 2009;**124**:e218-e226

[29] Lynch HJ, Wurtman RJ, Moskowitz MA, et al. Daily rhythm in human urinary melatonin. Science. 1975;**187**:169-171

[30] Tan DX, Reiter RJ, Manchester LC, et al. Chemical and physical properties and potential mechanisms: Melatonin as a broad spectrum antioxidant and free radical scavenger. Current Topics in Medicinal Chemistry. 2002;**2**:181-197

[31] Uchida K, Samejima M, Okabe A, et al. Neuroprotective effects of melatonin against anoxia/ aglycemia stress, as assessed by synaptic potentials and superoxide production in rat hippocampal slices. Journal of Pineal Research. 2004;**37**:215-222

[32] Welin AK, Svedin P, Lapatto R, et al. Melatonin reduces inflammation and cell death in white matter in the mid-gestation fetal sheep following umbilical cord occlusion. Pediatric Research. 2007;**61**:153-158

[33] Lee MY, Kuan YH, Chen HY, et al. Intravenous administration of melatonin reduces the intracerebral cellular inflammatory response following transient focal cerebral ischemia in rats. Journal of Pineal Research. 2007;**42**:297-309

[34] Reiter RJ, Calvo JR, Karbownik M, et al. Melatonin and its relation to the immune system and inflammation.

Annals of the New York Academy of Sciences. 2000;**917**:376-386

[35] Robertson NJ, Faulkner S, Fleiss B, et al. Melatonin augments hypothermic neuroprotection in a perinatal asphyxia model. Brain. 2013;**136**:90-105

[36] Boda M, Nemeth I, Boda D. The caffeine metabolic ratio as an index of xanthine oxidase activity in clinically active and silent celiac patients. Journal of Pediatric Gastroenterology and Nutrition. 1999;**29**:546-550

[37] Kaandorp JJ, Derks JB, Oudijk MA, et al. Antenatal allopurinol reduces hippocampal brain damage after acute birth asphyxia in late gestation fetal sheep. Reproductive Sciences. 2014;**21**:251-259

[38] Follett PL, Deng W, Dai W, et al. Glutamate receptor-mediated oligodendrocyte toxicity in periventricular leukomalacia: A protective role for topiramate. The Journal of Neuroscience. 2004;**24**:4412-4420

[39] Noh MR, Kim SK, Sun W, et al. Neuroprotective effect of topiramate on hypoxic ischemic brain injury in neonatal rats. Experimental Neurology. 2006;**201**:470-478

[40] Schubert S, Brandl U, Brodhun M, et al. Neuroprotective effects of topiramate after hypoxia ischemia in newborn piglets. Brain Research. 2005;**1058**:129-136

[41] Liu Y, Barks JD, Xu G, et al. Topiramate extends the therapeutic window for hypothermia-mediated neuroprotection after stroke in neonatal rats. Stroke. 2004;**35**:1460-1465

[42] Filippi L, Poggi C, la Marca G, et al. Oral topiramate in neonates with hypoxic ischemic encephalopathy treated with hypothermia: A safety study. The Journal of Pediatrics. 2010;**157**:361-366

[43] Baumert JH, Hein M, Hecker KE, et al. Autonomic cardiac control with xenon anaesthesia in patients at cardiovascular risk. British Journal of Anaesthesia. 2007;**98**:722-727

[44] Wappler F, Rossaint R, Baumert J, et al. Multicenter randomized comparison of xenon and isoflurane on left ventricular function in patients undergoing elective surgery. Anesthesiology. 2007;**106**:463-471

[45] Banks P, Franks NP, Dickinson R. Competitive inhibition at the glycine site of the N-methyl-D-aspartate receptor mediates xenon neuroprotection against hypoxia-ischemia. Anesthesiology. 2010;**112**:614-622

[46] Wilhelm S, Ma D, Maze M, et al. Effects of xenon on in vitro and in vivo models of neuronal injury. Anesthesiology. 2002;**96**:1485-1491

[47] Hobbs C, Thoresen M, Tucker A, et al. Xenon and hypothermia combine additively, offering long-term functional and histopathologic neuroprotection after neonatal hypoxia/ischemia. Stroke. 2008;**39**:1307-1313

[48] Chakkarapani E, Dingley J, Liu X, et al. Xenon enhances hypothermic neuroprotection in asphyxiated newborn pigs. Annals of Neurology. 2010;**68**:330-341

[49] Dalkara T, Yoshida T, Irikura K, et al. Dual role of nitric oxide in focal cerebral ischemia. Neuropharmacology. 1994;**33**:1447-1452

[50] Rao S, Lin Z, Drobyshevsky A, et al. Involvement of neuronal nitric oxide synthase in ongoing fetal brain injury following near-term rabbit hypoxia-ischemia. Developmental Neuroscience. 2011;**33**:288-298

[51] Drury PP, Davidson JO, van den Heuij LG, et al. Partial neuroprotection by nNOS inhibition during profound asphyxia in preterm fetal sheep. Experimental Neurology. 2013;**250**:1-21

[52] Grimm S. The ER–mitochondria interface: The social network of cell death. Biochimica et Biophysica Acta (BBA) - Molecular Cell Research. 2012;**1823**:327-334

[53] Wu G, Majewski J, Ege C, et al. Interaction between lipid monolayers and Poloxamer 188: An X-ray reflectivity and diffraction study. Biophysical Journal. 2005;**89**:3159-3173

[54] Firestone MA, Seifert S. Interaction of nonionic PEO-PPO Diblock copolymers with lipid bilayers. Biomacromolecules. 2005;**6**:2678-2687

[55] Shelat PB, Plant LD, Wang JC, et al. The membrane-active tri-block copolymer Pluronic F-68 profoundly rescues rat hippocampal neurons from oxygen–glucose deprivation-induced death through early inhibition of apoptosis. The Journal of Neuroscience. 2013;**33**:12287-12299

[56] Marks JD, Pan CY, Bushell T, et al. Amphiphilic, tri-block copolymers provide potent, membrane-targeted neuroprotection. FASEB Journal Express Article. 2001;**15**(6):1107-1109. DOI: 10.1096/fj.00-0547fje

[57] Marks JD, Doi A, Garcia AG, et al. Poloxamer 188, an amphiphilic tri-block co-polymer, provides profound hippocampal neuroprotection following transient global forebrain ischemia in the Mongolian gerbil. 2007 Neuroscience Meeting Planner. 2007

[58] Ballas SK, Files B, Luchtman-Jones L, et al. Safety of purified poloxamer 188 in sickle cell disease: Phase I study of a non-ionic surfactant in the management of acute chest syndrome. Hemoglobin. 2004;**28**:85-102

[59] Duvinage C, Millecamps S, Sagnier A, et al. One month intravenous toxicity studies of poloxamer 188 in male Sprague-Dawley rats and in beagle dogs. Toxicology Letters. 1996;**88**:101

[60] Erecinska M, Thoresen M, Silver IA. Effects of hypothermia on energy metabolism in mammalian central nervous system. Journal of Cerebral Blood Flow and Metabolism. 2003;**23**:513-530

[61] Girnsberg MD. Temperature influences on ischemic brain injury. In: Hsu CY, editor. Ischemic Stroke: From Basic Mechanism to New Drug Development. Vol. 16. Basel: Monogr Clin Neurosci. Karger; 1998. pp. 65-88

[62] Rincon F, Mayer SA. Therapeutic hypothermia for brain injury after cardiac arrest. Seminars in Neurology. 2006;**26**:387-395

[63] Berger C, Schabitz WR, Georgiadis D, et al. Effects of hypothermia on excitatory amino acids and metabolism in stroke patients: A micro-dialysis study. Stroke. 2002;**33**:519-524

[64] Hemmen TM, Lyden PD. Induced hypothermia for acute stroke. Stroke. 2007;**28**:794-799

Chapter 2

Ancillary Imaging Tests for Confirmation of Brain Death

Sudharsana Rao Ande and Jai Jai Shiva Shankar

Abstract

Brain death is an irreversible termination of functions of the entire brain including brain stem. The American Association of Neurology has defined brain death with three cardinal criteria, namely cessation of the functions of brain including brain stem, coma or unresponsiveness, and apnea. Ancillary testing is done in situations where clinical criteria of brain death cannot be determined by neurological examination or by apnea test. Ancillary tests for determining brain death can be primarily divided into two groups. One group includes tests that can test brain's electrical functions and the other group includes tests that can document cerebral blood flow in the brain on imaging. In this chapter, we present characteristics of the ideal ancillary test in the diagnosis of brain death and also describe various types of ancillary imaging tests used in the clinical setting for brain death determination and the merits and demerits associated with these techniques.

Keywords: brain death, ancillary imaging test, brainstem function, computed tomography, DSA, nuclear scintigraphy, CT perfusion (CTP), CT angiography (CTA), magnetic resonance imaging (MRI), magnetic resonance angiography (MRA), magnetic resonance perfusion (MRP)

1. Introduction

Brain death is defined as permanent cessation of all vital functions of the brain. It is principally established using clinical criteria including coma, absence of brain stem reflexes, and using apnea test. In Canada, two physicians must determine whether particular patient is brain dead or not [1, 2]. The criteria for declaring brain death includes deep unresponsive coma with established etiology, absence of reversible conditions [2]. Absence of brain stem reflexes includes absence of gag, cough, bilateral absence of corneal response, pupillary response to light and vestibule-ocular response, absence of respiratory efforts based on apnea test, and absence of confounding factors [2]. Ancillary imaging tests are necessary in situations when neurological examination or the apnea test cannot be performed or its validity comes into a question [3]. These situations include when patients have resuscitated shock, hypothermia, severe metabolic abnormalities, complex spinal reflexes, peripheral nerve or muscular dysfunctions, high cervical spine injury, craniofacial trauma or if the patient is on sedative drugs such as alcohol, barbiturates, sedatives, and hypnotics.

An ideal ancillary test should not have any false positive results. This is very important in brain death patients. If the ancillary test confirms death, when in fact, patient is not dead, is very dangerous and raises critical social, ethical and legal concerns. The main objective of the ancillary test would be to demonstrate the absence of cerebral electric activity or cerebral circulatory arrest [4]. Based on this, the first type assesses the electrical functions of the brain, and the other type analyses cerebral blood flow in the brain on imaging. Here, we provide description of cerebral blood flow imaging techniques and compare them.

2. Characteristics of ideal ancillary test for determining the brain death

Young and his colleagues described the attributes of an ideal ancillary test [5]. A reliable ancillary test should meet all the criteria mentioned below.

1. When the test confirms brain death, there should be no one that recovers or have the potential to recover. There should be no false positives.

2. The test should be independently sufficient enough to establish whether brain death is present or not.

3. The test should not be susceptible to external or internal confounding factors such as drug effects and metabolic disturbances.

4. The test should have standardized technology, technique, and classification of results.

5. The test should be inexpensive, safe, and readily applied. Testing should not be restricted to only few tertiary academic centers. It could be applied with any intensive care unit, and the technique should be mastered without difficulty.

3. Ancillary imaging tests used in brain death determination

3.1 Digital subtraction angiography (DSA)

This is considered the gold standard for ancillary imaging test. DSA is the first used modality for determining the cerebral blood flow. It is typically performed with a catheter tip in the aortic arch and contrast injection into each of the four arteries supplying the brain [3]. At least two injections, 20 min apart, must show an absence of filling of four arteries as their course becomes intracranial (**Figure 1**) [3, 6].

This test is capable of detecting dynamic blood flow in the arteries, veins, and capillaries. The criteria for brain death diagnosis using this method include no intracerebral filling at the level of entry into the skull of carotid or vertebral artery and filling of external carotid arteries. But this method does not have the spatial resolution to distinguish the blood flow in the different parts of the brain such as brainstem. Other disadvantages include transportation of patents to the angio suite; requires expert operator to perform; is invasive; and requires injection of contrast medium that may have a potential risk to the patients with kidney diseases. It can have "stasis filling" due to diffusion of contrast in the static column of blood, which can result in false negatives. Thus, it is an expensive procedure and not readily available in many hospitals and may not be easy to interpret in many healthcare facilities.

3.2 Nuclear scintigraphy

This is another gold standard ancillary imaging test for determination of brain death. In this technique, a gamma emitting radioactive tracer is intravenously

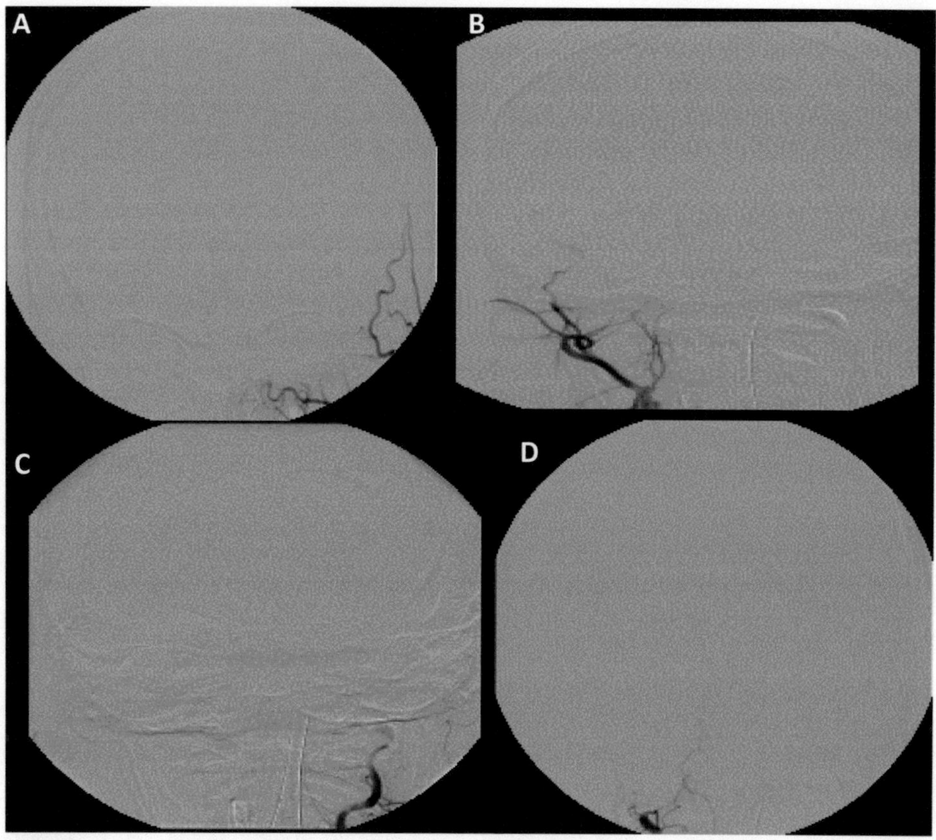

Figure 1.
Digital subtraction angiography image of a brain dead patient showing no intracranial filling on selective (A) left and (B) right common carotid artery as well as (C) left and (D) right vertebral artery angiograms. These show continued filling of the extracranial arteries including (A) left and (B) right external carotid arteries.

injected and is detected by a radio counter in the nuclear medicine. One of the radioactive tracers used is Tc99m-DTPA. After bolus intravenous injection of the tracer, brain vascular flow is estimated. DTPA does not have the ability to cross the intact blood brain barrier, so intracranial blood flow is seen in normal patients. However, Tc99m-DTPA tracer has low resolution for brain vascular flow [7]. There are two other radiopharmaceuticals, namely Tc99m-HMPAO (hexamethylpropyleneamine oxime) and Tc99m-ECD (ethyl cysteinate dimer) [8]. Both of them are brain specific, lipophilic and after intravenous injection, they cross the blood brain barrier. Because of this property, they are accumulated proportional to the blood flow in normal gray matter including brain cells of cerebrum, cerebellum, and brainstem [8]. So, it is not only blood flow but also brain parenchyma is seen in the normal functioning brain. In this method, radioactive isotope is injected 30 min after its reconstitution. Images are taken immediately after injection, after 30 min, and finally after 2 hours. If there is no blood flow, there is no accumulation of tracer in the brain and brain looks hollow, this phenomenon is known as "hollow skull" or "empty bulb" sign (**Figure 2**). These injected radioactive tracer compounds are safe to the patients because they do not interact with their medication and have no associated side effects [8].

Disadvantages of this technique is sometimes posterior fossa may be difficult to visualize, and uptake may be affected by hypothermia and barbiturates [3]. It does not have the spatial resolution to detect isolated brainstem activity. Other disadvantages include associated time delay and availability of this technique. Nuclear scintigraphy requires instrumentation, an experienced radiologist to interpret the test results, and the radioactive tracer used in this test is expensive and requires a trained pharmacist to reconstitute.

3.3 CT head

Computed tomography (CT) was introduced in 1970, since then it has revolutionized the assessment of head injuries including brain death [9]. It is fast, readily available, and requires no contrast medium. It is a standard imaging test for the patients admitted in the hospital because of brain injuries. Plain head CT scan can visualize brain tissue and lesion. It accurately diagnoses skull fractures, intracranial bleeds, brain contusions, and brain herniation. For diagnosis of brain death, a diffuse loss of gray-white mater differentiation needs to be established (**Figure 3**).

Plain head CT has several limitations in assessment of brain death. Plain head CT does not provide functional information of the brain and does not assess

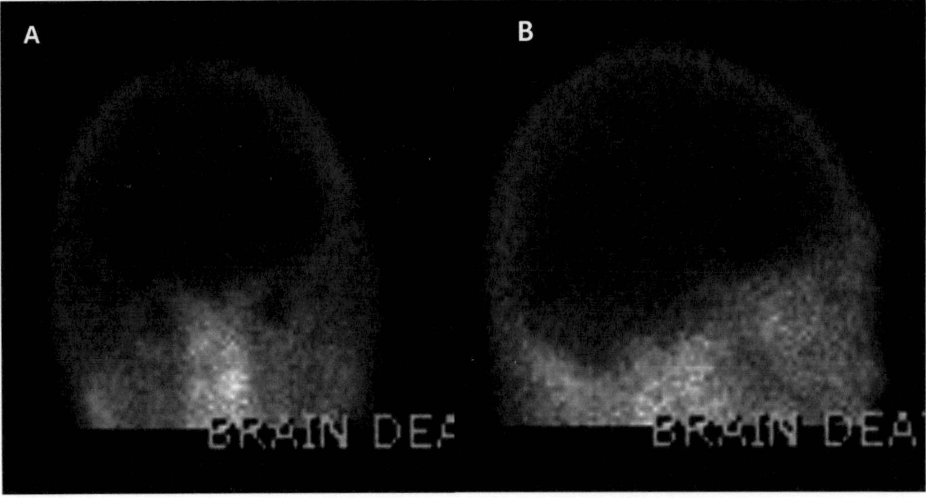

Figure 2.
"Hallow skull"/"empty bulb" sign shown in brain death patient using (A) AP and (B) lateral nuclear scintigraphy imaging. Flow and delayed imaging demonstrated no significant intracranial flow or parenchymal uptake.

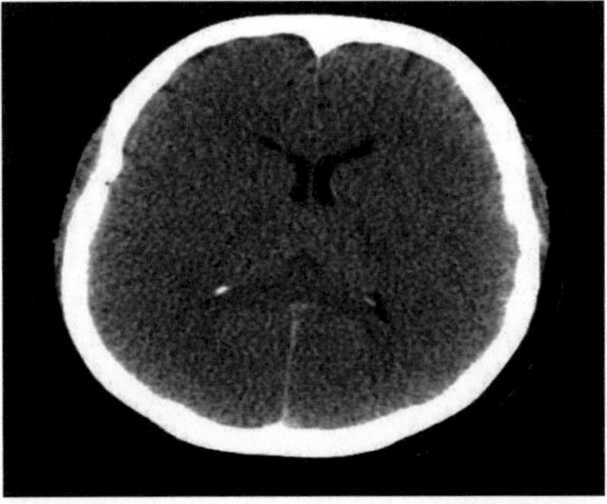

Figure 3.
Plain head CT image of a brain dead patient showing diffuse loss of gray-white mater differentiation.

intracranial blood flow. Diffuse loss of gray-white mater differentiation is likely a late phenomenon and the inter-rater reliability is poor [10].

Contrast enhanced CT of head can be acquired to assess brain blood flow but is delayed compared to CT angiography. Contrast-enhanced CT acquisition requires a delay of 5 min, whereas CT angiography requires only 12–16 seconds. This delay makes the contrast-enhanced CT highly susceptible to "stasis filling" of the brain blood vessels. Thus, plain head CT is not very reliable test in determining brain death.

3.4 Computed tomography angiography (CTA)

CTA is a valuable ancillary imaging technique for intracranial blood flow. CTA was first reported in 1998 as an ancillary test in diagnosing the brain death [11]. According to Dupas et al., in 14 patients who were diagnosed as brain dead using clinical criteria, the results were confirmed to have 100% sensitivity using CTA [11]. CTA is fast, non-invasive, technically noncomplicated, inexpensive, readily and widely available. It is perhaps the most widely available brain blood-flow test. CTA has a high spatiotemporal resolution and is relatively operator independent. Several European countries have adopted CTA as an ancillary test but not the United States [12, 13].

The technique of CTA involves rapid intravenous administration of iodinated contrast followed by volume scanning of the whole brain. For imaging of brain death at least two acquisitions should be performed, 60 seconds apart [9]. Others have proposed at least three acquisitions-arterial phase scanning after 20 seconds and venous phase scanning after 50–60 seconds [4].

Diagnostic criteria for brain death using CTA include lack of intracranial arterial contrast opacification. Lack of intracranial contrast opacification can be assessed by 4, 7, and 10 point scales. In 4 point scale, M4 (cortical) segments of middle cerebral artery (MCA) and intracerebral vein (ICV) are evaluated for contrast opacification [11]. The 7 point scale included evaluation of MCA-M4, anterior cerebral artery (ACA), ICV, and great cerebral vein (GCV) [14]. In the 10 point scale, all the seven segments of the 7 point scale plus posterior cerebral artery (PCA) and basilar artery are included [6]. In a recent study, Garret et al. assessed statistical performance of CTA in diagnosing brain death. For all the 18 patients included in the study, CTA had sensitivity of 75%, specificity of 100%, positive predictive value of 100%, and negative predictive value of 33% [15]. Another recent study from Macdonald et al. reported the diagnostic accuracy and inter-rater reliability of different ancillary imaging tests used for brain death in 74 patients. They showed that CTA along with CTP and radionuclide scan had a specificity and positive predictive value of 100% [10]. These results certainly add to the growing medical literature that supports the use of CTA as a reliable ancillary imaging test in confirming the brain death. However, systematic reviews do not support use of CTA as an ancillary imaging test for confirmation of brain death [16, 17].

The disadvantages of CTA are that this is not widely available as a bedside test and patient needs to be transported to imaging facility and this is challenging for an intensive care unit (ICU) patient. However, this can be obviated by the use of portable CT scanners in the future. CTA provides incomplete quantitative measurement of cerebral blood flow due predominantly of "stasis filling" (**Figure 4**). It is defined as delayed, weak persistent opacification of proximal cerebral arteries. This phenomenon causes a major problem in the development of reliable CTA protocol for the diagnosis of brain death [6]. There is also potential risk of damage to the organs of the brain death patients because of iodinated

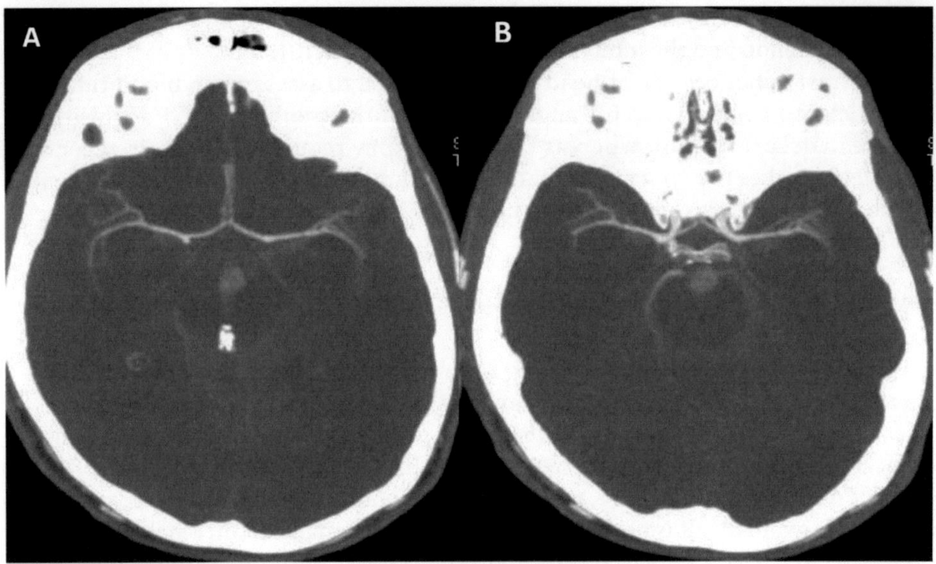

Figure 4.
Axial CTA images (A, B) in patient with clinically confirmed brain death show contrast opacification of bilateral internal carotid arteries, proximal branches of bilateral middle, and anterior cerebral arteries. None of the two images show opacification of M4 or cortical branches of middle cerebral arteries, distal anterior cerebral artery (ACA), internal and great cerebral vein. There is some opacification of only right posterior cerebral artery. There is continued filling of the extra cranial arteries.

contrast media used in CTA. However based on the volume of contrast used for CTA, this is rare or negligible [18, 19].

3.5 Computed tomography perfusion (CTP)

CTP is an advanced CT scan technique that provides both anatomical as well as functional information about the brain. CTP is useful in detecting perfusion even in small vessels such as arterioles, capillaries, and venules [20]. CTP is routinely used for evaluation of cerebral ischemia and vascularization of brain tumors and has the spatial resolution to quantify perfusion in any selected part of the brain [21, 22]. This imaging technique can help in calculation of cerebral blood flow (CBF) and cerebral blood volume (CBV). Normal CBF in the brain is 50–60 ml/100 mg/min and CTP can measure as low as 1.2 ml/100 mg/min [20]. CTP is very sensitive in detecting the blood flow and can detect decreased perfusion as low as 2–3% in CBF and 2% in CBV [23]. In CTP acquisition protocol, patients will undergo whole brain coverage with 80 kVp, 100 mAs resulting in a radiation dose of approximately CT dose index of 189.64 mGy [20]. A minimum scan duration of 60 seconds is recommended to reliably cover the venous phase of the circulation. A total of 40 ml nonionic iodinated contrast medium injected at the rate of 5 ml/seconds, followed by 40 ml of saline flush at the rate of 5 ml/seconds. Regular perfusion analysis is performed if intracranial arteries are seen on the source images [20]. Whole brain death could be seen as no intracranial CBF or CBV (**Figure 5**). Shankar et al. compared CTP and CTA derived from the CTP for confirmation of brain death in a retrospective review of 11 patients clinically suspected of brain death [20]. CTA showed a sensitivity of 72.7% for 7- and 4-point scales, 81.8% sensitivity for opacification of ICV, and 100% sensitivity for CTP scores in the brainstem [20]. They, for the first time, showed that CTP can be a valuable ancillary tool in early detection of brain death. Recently, Sawicki et al. tested the reliability and diagnostic accuracy of CTP over CTA in determining brain death [24]. For whole brain CTP, they also showed a sensitivity of 100% to confirm the diagnosis of brain death [24]. MacDonald et al. showed similar sensitivity [10].

CTP can also evaluate brain-stem specific CBF [10, 20]. The concept of isolated brainstem death was first proposed by Shankar et al. in clinically confirmed brain death patients (**Figure 6**) [20]. Exact pathophysiological mechanism behind isolated brainstem death is not yet known. This is described when in patients with

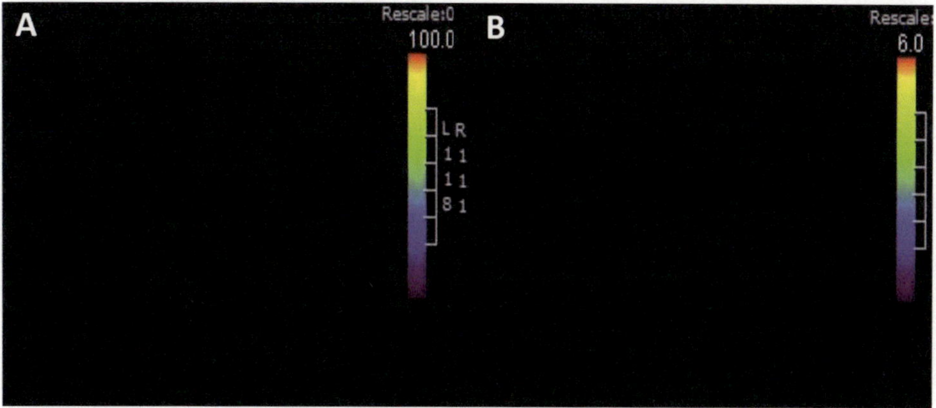

Figure 5.
CT perfusion showing no detectable cerebral blood flow (CBF) (A) and cerebral blood volume (CBV) (B) in the whole brain.

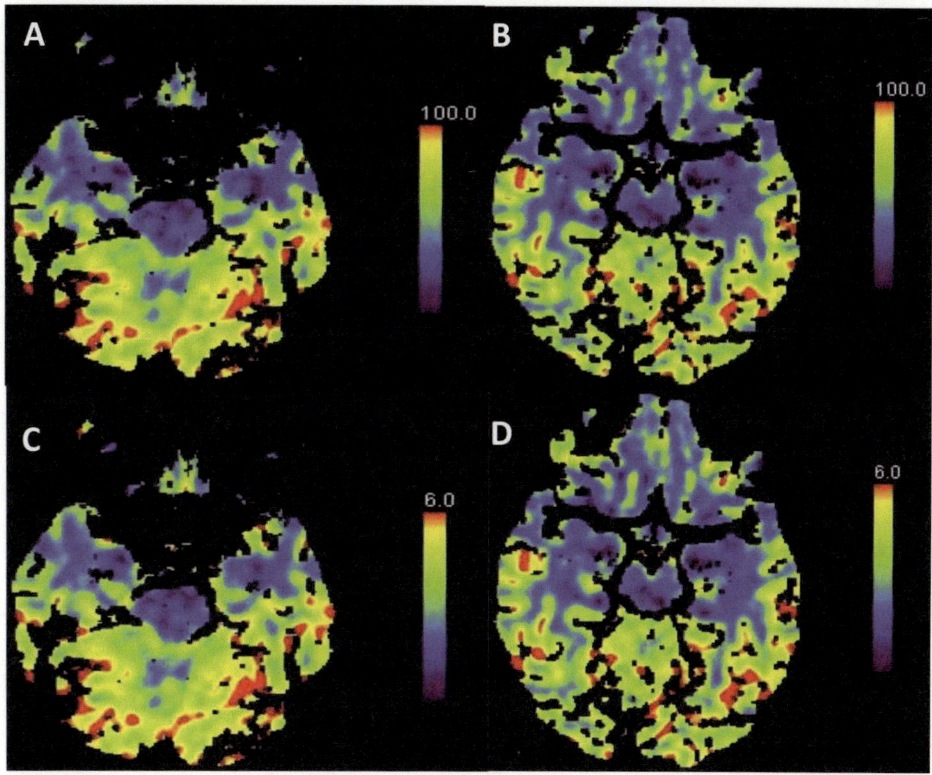

Figure 6.
CT perfusion showing matched defect on cerebral blood flow (CBF) (A and B) and cerebral blood volume (CBV) (C and D) maps in brainstem only. The supratentorial brain as well as cerebellum showed preserved CBF and CBV.

clinically confirmed brain death, there is presence of blood flow in the supratentorial brain and isolated absence of blood flow in the brainstem [10, 20]. Clinical examination does not differentiate between whole brain death and isolated brainstem death. CTP is the first imaging test reported to show the phenomenon of isolated brainstem death [10, 20]. It is suspected that isolated brainstem death is an earlier phenomenon in the process of brain death and may help early declaration of brain death [10]. However, the concept of brainstem death is debatable at the present time, and more studies are needed to establish this phenomenon.

Like CTA, CTP is a widely available tool and with the availability of automated software, CTP is relatively operator-independent [20]. The advantage of CTP is that it can be performed along with CTA. CTP has a presumed risk of contrast induced renal damage in the patients with kidney disease. But, based on the volume of contrast used for CTP, the chances of nephrotoxicity is very rare or negligible [18, 19].

3.6 Magnetic resonance imaging (MRI)

It is a reliable high-resolution imaging of brain and has been used for imaging for brain death. MRI has an advantage of not requiring nephrotoxic contrast material for demonstration of cerebral blood flow. It is noninvasive and accurate in identifying structural abnormalities in the brain. Common MRI findings in brain death patients are variable edema, diffuse cortical high signal intensity, diffuse cerebral white matter injury, and tonsillar herniation [25, 26]. Lovblad and colleagues demonstrated the usefulness of diffusion weighted imaging (DWI) in the diagnosis of brain death [27]. They reported that apparent diffusion coefficient (ADC) values are reduced in brain death patients when compared to the normal individuals [27]. Using DWI and ADC mapping, it is possible to identify areas of cytotoxic damage and ischemic damage [4]. However, this has not been accepted in the imaging guidelines for brain death. The major disadvantages of this method are the length of the scan time and obtaining MRI on ventilated patients as they may have several contraindications to MRI.

3.7 Magnetic resonance angiography (MRA)

It is a reliable test for cerebral blood flow [28] and can detect intracranial arterial blood flow and flow voids (**Figure 7**). However, MRA has not yet been proven as an ancillary test in assessing the brain death. Time of flight MRA is relatively immune to "stasis filling" when compared to CTA or DSA. Like any MRI, the patient needs

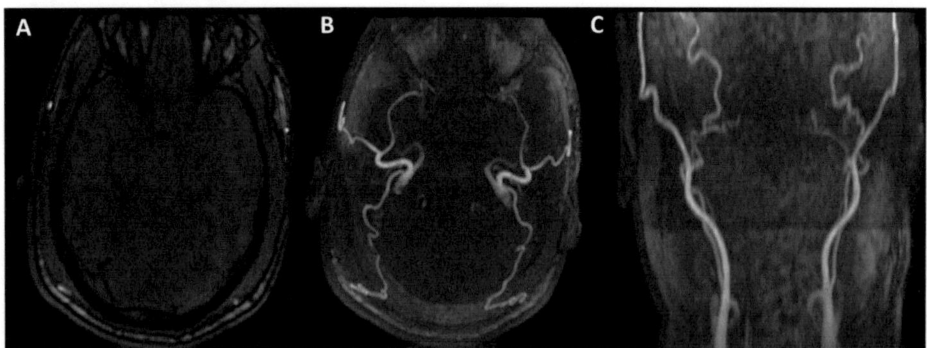

Figure 7.
Time of flight MR angiography image of a brain dead patient showed no intracranial flow but preserved extracranial flow on source image (A), axial (B), and coronal (C) maximum intensity projection images.

transportation to the radiology department, and the length of time for MRA is longer than that for CTA or CTP. There is requirement of having specialized critical care equipment in a scanner.

3.8 Magnetic resonance perfusion (MR perfusion)

MRP is noninvasive and can be used to detect intracranial arterial blood flow. It can also detect perfusion parameters of affected brain tissues such as cerebral blood flow and cerebral blood volume. There are not many reports in the literature that used MR perfusion as an ancillary imaging tool, and more research studies are needed to establish the reliability of this technique in the clinical setting.

4. Conclusions

For clinical confirmation of brain death, the three essential criteria are apnea, absence of brain stem reflexes, and coma. In situations where brain death cannot be confirmed by one of these clinical tests or there are uncertainties around the reliability of clinical examination, ancillary imaging techniques are required to confirm brain death. We describe different ancillary imaging tests commonly used and reported to confirm the brain death. More research is required to validate these tests to become gold standards in the clinical practice.

Conflict of interests

Jai Shankar is the co-PI of ongoing INDEX study for prospective evaluation of CT perfusion for confirmation of brain death.

Author details

Sudharsana Rao Ande and Jai Jai Shiva Shankar*
Division of Neuroradiology, Department of Radiology, University of Manitoba, Winnipeg, MB, Canada

*Address all correspondence to: shivajai1@gmail.com

References

[1] Heran MKS, Heran NS, Shemie SD. A review of ancillary tests in evaluating brain death. Canadian Journal of Neurological Sciences. 2008;**35**(4):409-419

[2] Shemie SD, Doig C, Dickens B, Byrne P, Wheelock B, Rocker G, et al. Severe brain injury to neurological determination of death: Canadian forum recommendations. Canadian Medical Association. 2006;**174**(6):S1-S13

[3] Busl KM, Greer DM. Pitfalls in the diagnosis of brain death. Neurocritical Care. 2009;**11**(2):276-287

[4] Sawicki M, Wojczal J, Birkenfeld B, Cyrylowski L. Brain death imaging. In: Saba L, Raz E, editors. Neurovascular Imaging. New York, NY: Springer; 2014. pp. 1-33. Available from: http://link.springer.com/10.1007/978-1-4614-9212-2_26-1

[5] Young GB, Shemie SD, Doig CJ, Teitelbaum J. Brief review: The role of ancillary tests in the neurological determination of death. Canadian Journal of Anesthesia. 2006;**53**(6):620-627

[6] Sawicki M, Bohatyrewicz R, Safranow K, Walecka A, Walecki J, Rowinski O, et al. Dynamic evaluation of stasis filling phenomenon with computed tomography in diagnosis of brain death. Neuroradiology. 2013;**55**(9):1061-1069

[7] Munari M, Zucchetta P, Carollo C, Gallo F, De Nardin M, Marzola MC, et al. Confirmatory tests in the diagnosis of brain death: Comparison between SPECT and contrast angiography. Critical Care Medicine. 2005;**33**(9):2068-2073

[8] Zuckier LS, Kolano J. Radionuclide studies in the determination of brain death: Criteria, concepts, and controversies. Seminars in Nuclear Medicine. 2008;**38**(4):262-273

[9] Rosenblum ML, Hoff JT, Norman D, Weinstein PR, Pitts L. Decreased mortality from brain abscesses since advent of computerized tomography. Journal of Neurosurgery. 1978;**49**(5):658-668

[10] MacDonald D, Stewart-Perrin B, Shankar JJS. The role of neuroimaging in the determination of brain death. Journal of Neuroimaging. 2018;**28**(4):374-379

[11] Dupas B, Gayet-Delacroix M, Villers D, Antonioli D, Veccherini MF, Soulillou JP. Diagnosis of brain death using two-phase spiral CT. American Journal of Neuroradiology. 1998;**19**(4):641-647

[12] Wijdicks EFM. Brain death worldwide: Accepted fact but no global consensus in diagnostic criteria. Neurology. 2002;**58**(1):20-25

[13] Beltramello A, Casartelli Liviero M, Bernardi B, Causin F, Di Paola F, Muto M, et al. Computed tomography angiography: A double step methodology in brain death confirmation. Minerva Anestesiologica. 2014;**80**(7):862-863

[14] Leclerc X, Taschner CA, Vidal A, Strecker G, Savage J, Gauvrit JY, et al. The role of spiral CT for the assessment of the intracranial circulation in suspected brain-death. Journal of Neuroradiology. 2006;**33**(2):90-95

[15] Garrett MP, Williamson RW, Bohl MA, Bird CR, Theodore N. Computed tomography angiography as a confirmatory test for the diagnosis of brain death. Journal of Neurosurgery. 2018;**128**(2):639-644

[16] Kramer AH, Roberts DJ. Computed tomography angiography in the

diagnosis of brain death: A systematic review and meta-analysis. Neurocritical Care. 2014;**21**(3):539-550

[17] Taylor T, Dineen RA, Gardiner DC, Buss CH, Howatson A, Pace NL. Computed tomography (CT) angiography for confirmation of the clinical diagnosis of brain death. Cochrane Database of Systematic Reviews. 2014;**3**:CD009694

[18] Hopyan JJ, Gladstone DJ, Mallia G, Schiff J, Fox AJ, Symons SP, et al. Renal safety of CT angiography and perfusion imaging in the emergency evaluation of acute stroke. American Journal of Neuroradiology. 2008;**29**(10):1826-1830

[19] Krol AL, Dzialowski I, Roy J, Puetz V, Subramaniam S, Coutts SB, et al. Incidence of radiocontrast nephropathy in patients undergoing acute stroke computed tomography angiography. Stroke. 2007;**38**(8):2364-2366

[20] Shankar JJS, Vandorpe R. CT perfusion for confirmation of brain death. American Journal of Neuroradiology. 2013;**34**(6):1175-1179

[21] Shankar JJS, Woulfe J, Silva VD, Nguyen TB. Evaluation of perfusion CT in grading and prognostication of high-grade gliomas at diagnosis: A pilot study. American Journal of Roentgenology. 2013;**200**(5):W504-W509

[22] Shankar JJS, Langlands G, Doucette S, Phillips S. CT perfusion in acute stroke predicts final infarct volume-inter-observer study. Canadian Journal of Neurological Sciences. 2016;**43**(1):93-97

[23] Uwano I, Kudo K, Sasaki M, Christensen S, Østergaard L, Ogasawara K, et al. CT and MR perfusion can discriminate severe cerebral hypoperfusion from perfusion absence: Evaluation of different commercial software packages by using digital phantoms. Neuroradiology. 2012;**54**(5):467-474

[24] Sawicki M, Sołek-Pastuszka J, Chamier-Ciemińska K, Walecka A, Bohatyrewicz R. Accuracy of computed tomographic perfusion in diagnosis of brain death: A prospective cohort study. Medical Science Monitor. 2018;**24**:2777-2785

[25] Ishii K, Onuma T, Kinoshita T, Shiina G, Kameyama M, Shimosegawa Y. Brain death: MR and MR angiography. American Journal of Neuroradiology. 1996;**17**(4):731-735

[26] Karantanas AH, Hadjigeorgiou GM, Paterakis K, Sfiras D, Komnos A. Contribution of MRI and MR angiography in early diagnosis of brain death. European Radiology. 2002;**12**(11):2710-2716

[27] Lövblad KO, Bassetti C, Basssetti C. Diffusion-weighted magnetic resonance imaging in brain death. Stroke. 2000;**31**(2):539-542

[28] Drake M, Bernard A, Hessel E. Brain death. The Surgical Clinics of North America. 2017;**97**(6):1255-1273

Chapter 3

Nonconvulsive Status Epilepticus and Coma

Demet Ilhan Algın, Gülgun Uncu, Demet Ozbabalık Adapınar and Oğuz Osman Erdinç

Abstract

Nonconvulsive status epilepticus (NCSE) is common in patients with coma with a prevalence between 5 and 48%. Nonconvulsive status epilepticus (NCSE) is an electroclinical state associated with an altered mental status (AMS) but lacking convulsive motor activity. It is difficult to diagnose in the obtunded/comatose patients. Such patients have often other serious medical conditions, and the diagnosis of NCSE is frequently delayed in these patients. Diagnosing NCSE demands a high degree of clinical suspicion and for that reason likely remains under-recognized. The most important question, however, is whether the treatment of NCSE in coma improves the outcome of these patients or not. In this review, we aimed to summarize the EEG patterns in NCSE to further delineate the borders between comatose forms of NCSE and coma-epileptiform discharges and to evaluate modified EEG criteria for NCSE in a coma.

Keywords: coma, nonconvulsive status epilepticus (NCSE), EEG, periodic discharges, consciousness

1. Introduction

Coma is the disorder of consciousness because of the damage to diffused bilateral cerebral hemisphere corte or ascending reticular activation system (ARAS) [1].

This neural network starts from the dorsal part of the upper pons, continues in the mesencephalon, connects to the thalamus and diffuses widely from there to both hemispheres. In addition, ARAS is associated with some nuclei in the pons and mesencephalon, the posterior hypothalamus, and the basal forebrain. Communication in this network is established through neurotransmitters such as acetylcholine, noradrenaline, serotonin and dopamine [2]. Structural or biochemical damage or disruption of this neural network may cause unconsciousness. The most severe picture in the spectrum of consciousness disorders is coma. In a comatose patient, alertness and awareness are completely lost. Many causes of both intracranial and systemic origin can cause coma. In order to begin specific treatment as soon as possible, the underlying cause of the coma should be established as quickly as possible. For this purpose, the patient should be systematically approached and the possible causes of the mechanism should be considered in five major categories [3]:

1. Unilateral hemispheric mass lesions compressing diencephalon or brain stem.

2. Bilateral hemispheric lesions affecting the reticular formation and thalamocortical cycle fibers at thalamus level.

3. Infratentorial lesions that compress or damage the reticular formation in the brain system.

4. Diffuse lesions affecting the physiological function of the brain.

5. Psychiatric conditions mimicking coma.

The evaluation of coma patients falls within the responsibility of physicians working in many disciplines. Detecting the cause of the coma requires detailed investigation and deductive effort. The physician should consider the patient as a whole and be able to synthesize the information obtained from history, examination and diagnostic tools and theoretical information.

2. Nonconvulsive status epilepticus

Nonconvulsive status epilepticus (NCSE) which has higher morbidity and mortality is a treatable disorder when diagnosed properly. NCSE has special symptoms such as unexplained confusion or coma or vegetative status and aura which can distinguish from the normal conditions. NCSE is a continuous seizure activity with a minimum duration of 10–30 min on EEG [4]. In previous studies used different EEG criteria to identify the NCSE patients, the prevalence of NCSE ranges from 5 to 48% and the actual prevalence of NCSE is still unknown [5].

B Without prominent motor symptoms (i.e., nonconvulsive SE, NCSE)

B-1 NCSE with coma (including so-called subtle SE)

B-2 NCSE without coma

B-2.a Generalized

B-2aa: Typical absence status

B-2ab:Atypical absence status

B-2ac:Myoclonic absence status

B-2b. Focal

B-2ba: Without impairment of conciousness (aura continua, with autonomic, sensory, visual, olfactory, gustatory, emotional/psychic/experiential, or auditory symptoms)

B-2bb: Aphasic status

B-2bc: With impaired consciousness

B-2c. Unknown whether focal or generalized (Autonomic SE)

B-2ca:Autonomic SE

Table 1.
New ILAE classification of NCSE axis 1.

The new ILAE classification is based on 4 axes 1 being the semiology (**Table 1**); axis 2 is the etiology; axis 3 is EEG correlates, and axis 4 is the age of the patient. This concept takes account of the requirements for a classification supporting a clinical diagnosis, enabling research through standardization while ensuring an individualized treatment concept for the patient [6, 7].

Clinical evidence may vary greatly in NCSE. Negative and positive symptoms can be evaluated into two groups. Negative symptoms are anorexia, aphasia/mutism, amnesia, catatonia, coma, lethargy and negative symptoms are agitation, aggression, automatisms, twinkle, crying, delirium, echolalia, laughing, nausea-vomiting, nystagmus-eye deviation, perseveration, anxiety and psychosis [8]. Nonconvulsive status epilepticus is a treatable neurologic emergency when it is diagnosed properly. Diagnostic criteria depend on clinical status, EEG findings and response to treatment. During the initial evaluation, EEG recording is crucial for patients with acute confusion [6].

Although the etiologies of NCSE and coma intersect, NCSE is a distinct clinical picture and an electroclinic condition without convulsive motor activity. Diagnosis is difficult in a comatose patient. The diagnosis of NCSE is often delayed in those patients. Clinically, a high degree of suspicion is required for diagnosis. Ictal-interictal discrimination of activity on EEG is difficult despite the newly defined criteria and these criteria have practical application difficulties. Another important issue is how aggressive treatment of NCSE in comatose patients should be, because the positive or negative effect of NCSE treatment on the prognosis of those patients is not well known. A distinction should be made between patients with coma or other severe disorders and those with really epileptic mechanisms and treatment should be decided accordingly. Specific EEG patterns are not seen in a coma [9].

2.1 EEG patterns in comatose patients

2.1.1 Intermittent rhythmic delta activity

Among EEG findings in encephalopathy, intermittent rhythmic delta activity (IRDA) is considered to lie at the milder end of the spectrum of coma EEG patterns. IRDA may appear in patients who are awake or who are mildly lethargic or stuporous; IRDA patterns are not associated with deeply comatose states. IRDA tends to occur in the frontal regions in adults (frontal intermittent rhythmic delta activity, or FIRDA) and in the occipital regions in (occipital intermittent rhythmic delta activity, or OIRDA) [10].

2.1.2 Prolonged bursts of slow-wave activity

Prolonged bursts of slow-wave activity can occur in a variety of etiologies in coma. They are most often diffuse but can also be lateralized without any spatiotemporal evolution [11].

2.1.3 Stimulus-induced rhythmic, periodic, or ictal discharges (SIRPIDs)

Stimulus-induced rhythmic, periodic, or ictal discharges (SIRPIDs) are a relatively common phenomenon found on prolonged electroencephalogram (EEG) monitoring that captures state changes and stimulation of comatose patients. Common causes include hypoxic injury, traumatic brain injury, and hemorrhage and toxic-metabolic disturbances [12, 13].

2.1.4 Generalized periodic and rhythmic discharges

Generalized periodic discharges (**Figure 1**) (GPDs) with a triphasic morphology have been associated with nonepileptic encephalopathies.

2.1.5 Lateralized periodic discharges

PLEDs (**Figure 2**) are usually associated with obtundation in 95% of patients, focal seizures and focal neurological signs may occur in 80%, and *Epilepsia partialis continua* in 30% of the patients [14, 15].

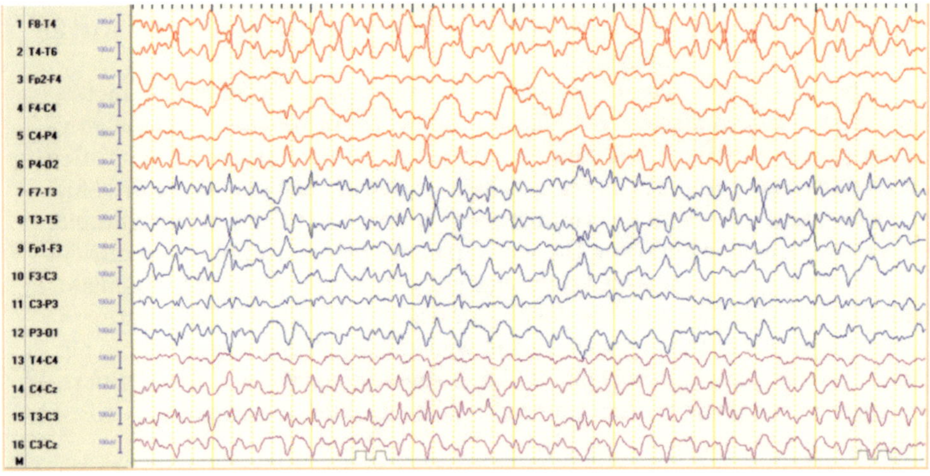

Figure 1.
A 45-year female patient coma due to intoxication with olanzapine continuous very regularly generalized 2–3/s spike and sharp wave activities.

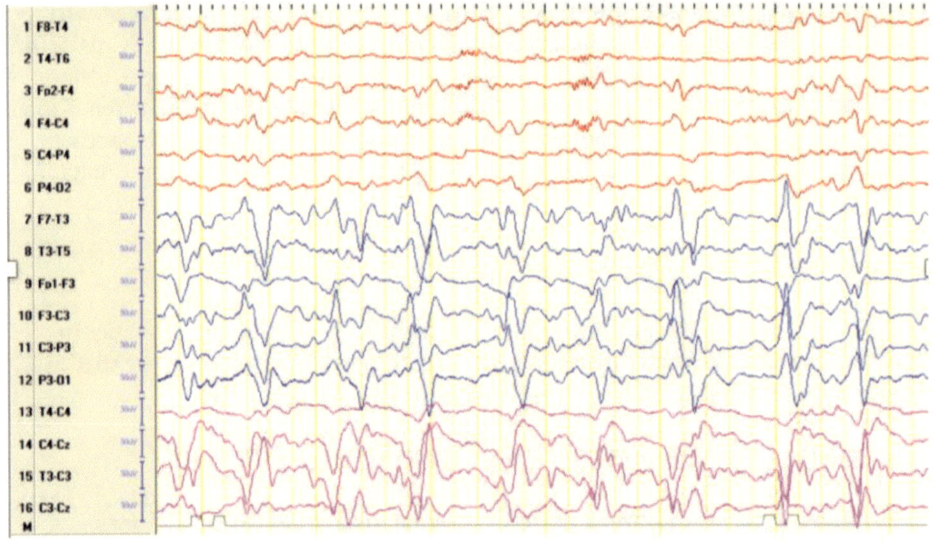

Figure 2.
A 40-year female, mentally retarded and epileptic patient admitted to our clinic with psychosis and diagnosed as limbic encephalitis. Lateralized periodic discharges left hemisphere. Flat periods with 1- to 2-second duration.

2.1.6 Triphasic waves (TWs)

Triphasic waves (**Figure 3**) are periodic and generalized, typically frontally predominant and not always epileptiform in appearance. This pattern can occur in any toxic-metabolic or structural encephalopathy although the early descriptions associated its presence to hepatic encephalopathy [16, 17].

2.1.7 Burst suppression patterns

Burst-suppression (**Figure 4**) in the electroencephalogram (EEG) is characterized by high amplitude events (bursts) alternated by periods of low or absent activity (suppressions). This pattern can be physiological, for instance during early development, or pathological, for example in almost half of comatose patients

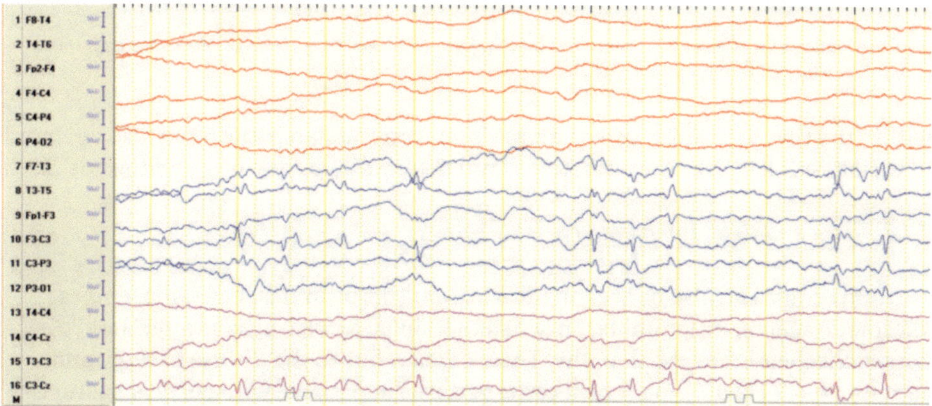

Figure 3.
A 61-year female patient, comatose state, had left-sided craniotomy after glioblastoma; EEG prominent in the left frontocentral region sharp waves with triphasic appearance.

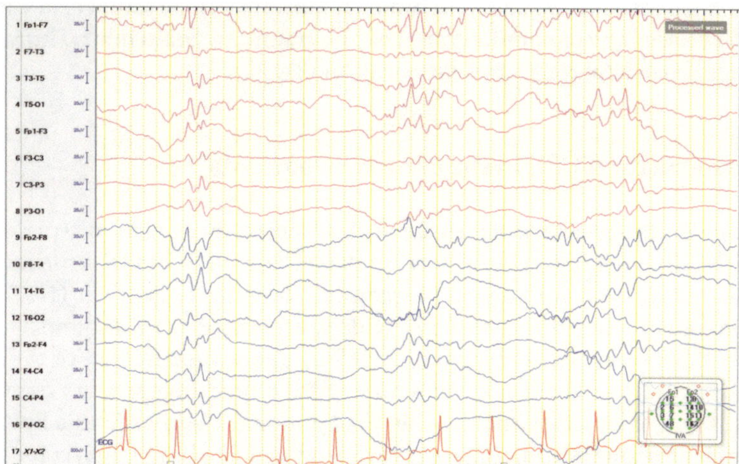

Figure 4.
A 70-year male patient, coma after cardiac arrest; EEG shows burst suppression pattern with bursts of mixed frequencies and interposed spikes and sharp waves. No response to treatment and died 7 days later.

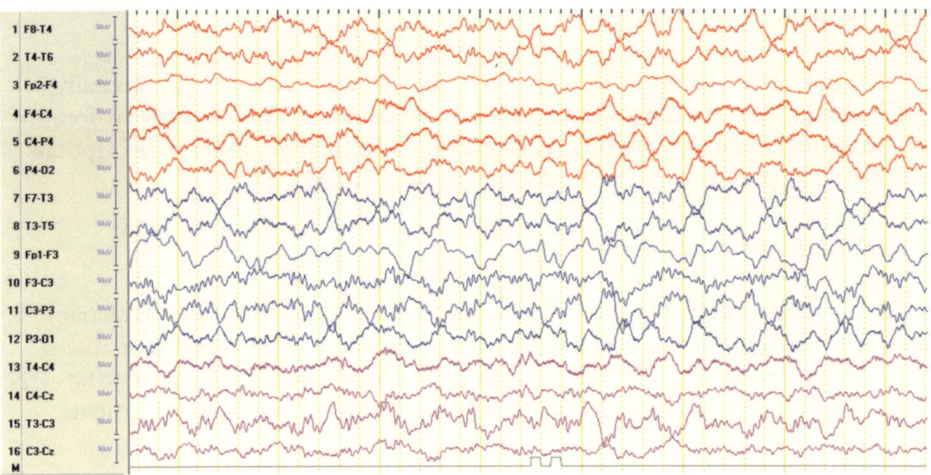

Figure 5.
A 45-year male patient, coma after traumatic brain injury; EEG shows 2-3 Hz delta slow waves with spindle prominent in the left frontocentral region.

within the first 48 h after cardiac arrest Burst suppression pattern can also be found in various etiologies (structural, toxic, and metabolic) or during hypothermia [18].

2.1.8 Alpha and theta coma patterns

Alpha coma can also be seen in intoxication (barbiturates, benzodiazepines, anesthetic agents, imipramine), brainstem lesions, locked-in syndrome and hypoxic-ischemic encephalopathy. Theta coma refers to the diffuse background activity of 4–7 Hz in coma. Theta coma patterns in patients with cortical dysfunction, such as in dementia or mild to moderate encephalopathy [19, 20].

2.1.9 Spindle coma patterns

Spindle coma patterns (**Figure** 5) in spindles, slow activity and K-complexes. They have been initially described in brain trauma but can be found also with other etiologies The etiology of spindle coma may be traumatic brain injury, intracerebral hemorrhage, post-ictal stages and intoxication [21, 22].

3. EEG criteria for NCSE in the comatose patients

Various EEG criteria have been used in previous studies to identify patients in comatose-NCSE, yielding a prevalence between 5 and 48%, but the true incidence of NCSE in coma is still not known. Nonconvulsive status epilepticus (NCSE) is a neurological emergency that is seen in a wide spectrum of cases. Diagnosis cannot be made without electroencephalography (EEG) due to the diversity of the clinical picture and the impaired consciousness due to the underlying primary damage, especially in intensive care patients. 4. In the London-Innsbruck Status Epilepticus meeting, the previous terminology was reviewed and Salzburg Criteria for the diagnosis of NCSE by Leitinger et al. reported [23–26] (**Table 2**).

In comatose patients, epileptiform discharges faster than 2.5 Hz or generalized periodic discharges (GPDs), lateralized periodic discharges (LPDs) and continuous 2/s GPDs with triphasic morphology of less than 2.5 Hz, as well as rhythmic

Patients without known epileptic encephalopathy
• EDs > 2.5 Hz, or
• EDs ≤ 2.5Hz or rhythmic delta/theta activity (>0.5 Hz) AN done of the following:
- EEG and clinical improvement after IV AEDs, or
- Subtle clinical ictal phenomena, or
- Typical spatiotemporal evolution
Patients with known epileptic encephalopathy
• Increase in prominence or frequency when compared with baseline with
• Improvement of clinical and EEG features with IV AEDs
*If EEG improvement without clinical improvement, or if fluctuation without definite evolution, this should be considered possible NCSE
**Incrementing onset (increase in voltage and change in frequency), or evolution in pattern (change in frequency N1 Hz or change in location), or decrementing termination (voltage or frequency)
EDs: epileptiform discharges (spikes, polyspikes, sharp waves, and sharp-and-slow-wave complexes)
IV AEDs: intravenous antiepileptic drugs

** Typical spatiotemporal evolution.*

Table 2.
The Salzburz consensus criteria for nonconvulsive stress epilepticus (NCSE).

discharges (RDs) faster than 0.5 Hz were also taken into consideration as NCSE if they responded to benzodiazepine treatment with improvement in the EEG or mental status of patient (**Figure 6**) [26, 27].

NCSE with coma can be accompanied by generalized epileptiform discharges (coma-GED) and coma with lateralized epileptiform discharges (coma-LED). Etiologic factors and EEG patterns found in coma-GED and coma-LED are given in [19, 28] (**Table 3**).

4. Conclusion

NCSE is a disorder comprising a broad clinical spectrum that requires characteristic electroencephalographic changes to confirm the correct diagnosis. NCSE is an under-recognized cause of coma and traditionally involves the clinical picture of an altered mental status with diminished responsiveness, a diagnostic EEG and often a response to antiepileptic therapy [29].

Mortality in nonconvulsive status epilepticus can be seen in 18–25%, and in severe patients with systemic disease followed by intensive care, this rate can increase to 50–52% [24]. It is important to decide how aggressive the treatment of NCSE in a coma should be. A distinction should be made between patients in coma and other severe illnesses and those in which epileptic mechanisms actually play a role, and treatment should be guided accordingly [30].

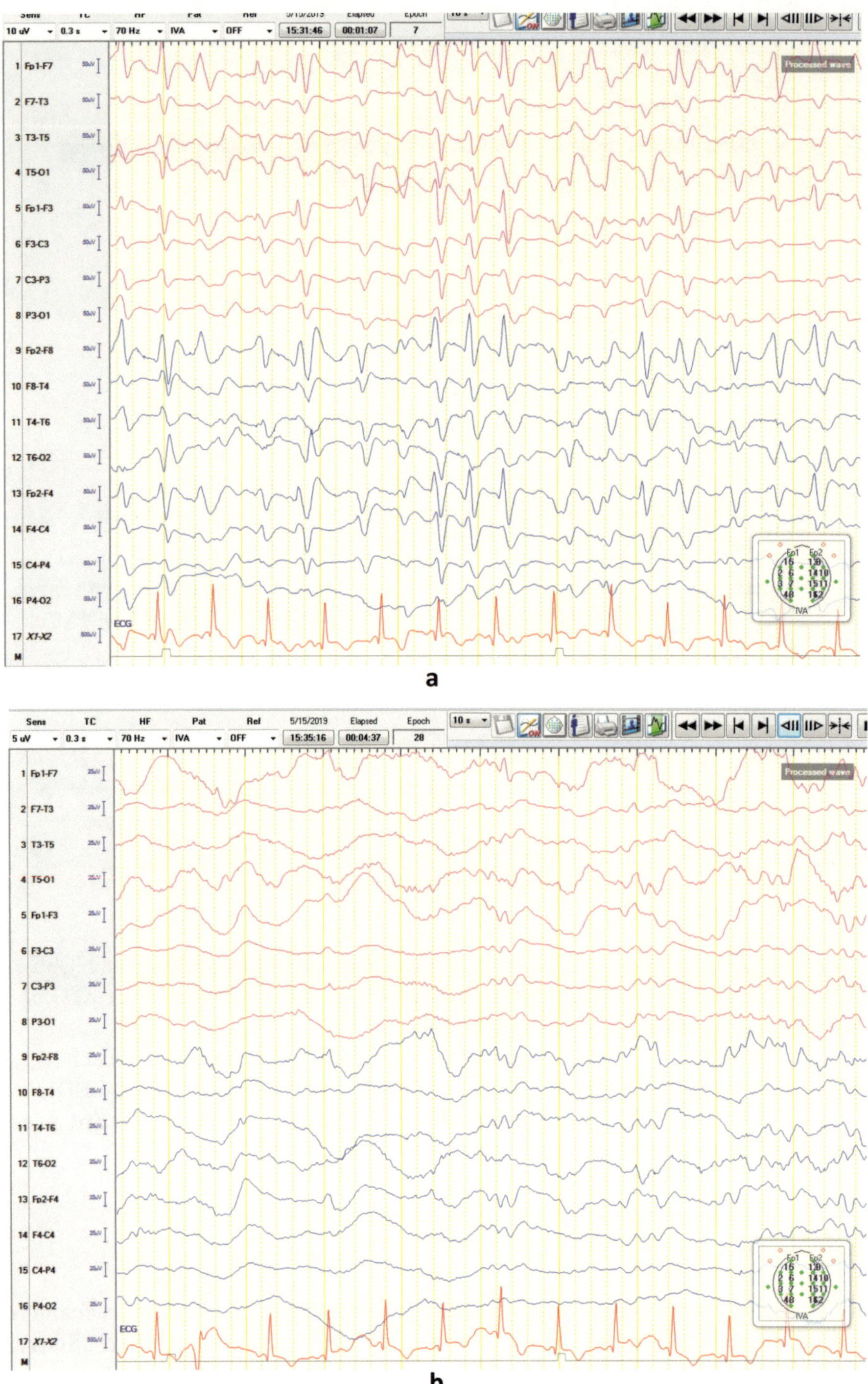

Figure 6.
(a) A 62-year female patient with breast cancer; confused; no abnormal movements; EEG shows repetitive generalized, >2.5/s spikes and slow waves with triphasic appearance. (b) Improvement of level of consciousness and EEG features following diazepam 10 mg IV.

Prognosis is better in patients with a history of epilepsy and prognosis in acutely symptomatic patients is related to the underlying disease. Convulsive and NCSE in patients with stroke, subarachnoid hemorrhage and traumatic brain injury worsen the prognosis by acting synergistically with acute brain pathology [31, 32].

	Etiology	EEG pattern
Coma-GED	Diffuse primary or secondary brain disturbances (anoxic, toxic, metabolic, infectious, degenerative) Space-occupying lesions with brainstem compression (direct or due to tentorial herniation) Known epilepsies?	Continuous generalized spiking Periodic spiking Burst suppression pattern in different variations
Coma-LED	Focal brain lesions (in most cases acutely acquired) In rare cases diffuse abnormalities (aminophylline intoxication, some forms of diabetic coma) Known epilepsies?	Continuous focal spiking PLEDs Bi-PLEDS Unilateral burst suppression pattern Unilateral triphasic waves
BI-PLED, bilateral periodic epileptiform discharges, GEDs, generalized epileptiform discharges; LED, lateralized epileptiform discharges; PLED, periodic epileptiform discharges.		

Table 3.
Etiologic factors and EEG pattern in comatose NCSE.

NCSE is a neurological emergency that can be treated if diagnosed properly. Diagnostic criteria depend on clinical status, EEG findings and response to treatment. EEG imaging is crucial for patients with acute confusion during the initial evaluation [33].

Acknowledgements

We would like to thank Neutec company for its support in publishing this section.

Author details

Demet Ilhan Algın[1], Gülgun Uncu[2*], Demet Ozbabalık Adapınar[3]
and Oğuz Osman Erdinç[1]

1 Department of Neurology, Faculty of Medicine, Eskişehir Osmangazi University, Eskişehir, Turkey

2 Department of Neurology, Eskişehir City Hospital, Eskişehir, Turkey

3 Department of Neurology, Eskişehir Acıbadem Hospital, Eskişehir, Turkey

*Address all correspondence to: drgulguncu@gmail.com

References

[1] Posner J, Saper C, Schiff N. Plum and Posner's Diagnosis of Stupor and Coma. 4th ed. Oxford Unıversity Press; 2007

[2] Felten DL, Jozefowicz RF. Brainstem and cerebellum. In: Netter's Atlas of Human Neuroscience. Icon Learning Systems LLC; 2003

[3] Wijdicks E. Comatose. In: The Practice of Emergency and Critical Care Neurology. Oxford University Press; 2010

[4] Altindag E, Okudan ZV, Özkan ST, KrespiY,BaykanB.Electroencephalographic patterns recorded by continuous EEG monitoring in patients with change of consciousness in the neurological intensive care unit. Archives of Neuropsychiatry. 2016

[5] Towne AR, Waterhouse EJ, Boggs JG, et al. Prevalence of nonconvulsive status epilepticus in comatose patients. Neurology. 2000;**54**:340-345

[6] Rüegg S. Nonconvulsive status epilepticus in adults: Types, pathophysiology, epidemiology, etiology, and diagnosis. Neurology International Open. 2017;**01**(03):E189-E203. DOI: 10.1055/s-0043-103383

[7] Rüegg S. Non-convulsive status epilepticus in adults: An overview. Schweizer Archiv für Neurologie und Psychiatrie. 2008;**159**:53-83

[8] Brophy GM, Bell R, Claassen J, Alldredge B, Beleck TP, Glauser T, et al. Guidelines for the evaluation and management of status epilepticus. Neurocritical Care. 2012;**17**:3-23

[9] Bauer G, Trinka E. Nonconvulsive status epilepticus and coma. Epilepsia. 2010;**51**:177-119

[10] Husain AM. Electroence phalographic assessment of coma. Journal of Clinical Neurophysiology. 2006;**23**(3):208-220

[11] Kubicki S, Rieger H. The EEG during acute intoxication with hypnotics. Electroencephalography and Clinical Neurophysiology. 1968;**25**(1):94

[12] Johnson EL, Kaplan PW, Ritzi EK. Stimulus-induced rhythmic, periodic, or Ictal Dıscharges (SIRPIDSs). Journal of Clinical Neurophysiology. 2018;**35**:229-233

[13] Hirsch LJ, Claassen J, Mayer SA, EmersonRG.Stimulus-inducedrhythmic, periodic, or ictal discharges (SIRPIDs): A common EEG phenomenon in the critically ill. Epilepsia. 2004;**45**:109-123

[14] Chatrian GE, Shaw CM, Leffman H. The significance of periodic lateralized epileptiform dischages in EEG: An electrographic, clinical and pathological study. Electroencephalography and Clinical Neurophysiology. 1964;**17**:177-193

[15] Gandelman-Marton R, Rabey JM, Flechter S. Periodic lateralized epileptiform discharges multiple sclerosis: A case report. Journal of Clinical Neurophysiology. 2003;**20**(2):117-121

[16] Brigo F, Storti M. Triphasic waves. American Journal of Electroneurodiagnostic Technology. 2011;**51**:16-25

[17] Brenner RP, Schaul N. Periodic EEG patterns: Classification, clinical correlation and pathophysiology. Journal of Clinical Neurophysiology. 1990;**7**:249-267

[18] Hofmeijer J, Tiepkema-Cloostermans MC, van Putten MJ. Burst-suppression with identical bursts: A distinct EEG pattern with poor outcome in postanoxic

coma. Clinical Neurophysiology. 2014;(5):947-954

[19] Kaplan PW, Genoud D, Ho TW, et al. Etiology, neurologic correlations, and prognosis in alpha coma. Clinical Neurophysiology. 1999;**110**:205-213

[20] Berkhoff M, Donati F, Bassetti C. Postanoxic alpha (theta) coma: A reappraisal of its prognostic significance. Clinical Neurophysiology. 2000;**111**:297-304

[21] Coma BG, Death B. In: Niedermeyer E, Lopez Da Silva F, editors. Electro-Encephalography: Basic Principles, Clinical Applications, and Related Fields. 4th ed. Baltimore: Williams and Wilkins; 1999. pp. 459-475

[22] Sutter R, Kaplan PW. Electroencephalographic patterns in coma: When things slow down. Epileptologie. 2012;**29**:201-209

[23] Hirsch LJ, Brenner RP, Drislane FW, So E, Kaplan PW, Jordan KG, et al. The ACNS subcommittee on research terminology for continuous EEG monitoring: Proposed standardized terminology for rhythmic and periodic EEG patterns encountered in critically ill patients. Journal of Clinical Neurophysiology. 2005;**22**(2):128-135

[24] Hirsch LJ, LaRoche SM, Gaspard N, Gerard E, Svoronos A, Herman ST, et al. American clinical neurophysiology Society's standardized critical care EEG terminology: 2012 version. Journal of Clinical Neurophysiology. 2013;**30**(1):1-27

[25] Leitinger M, Beniczky S, Rohracher A, Gardella E, Kalss G, Qerama E, et al. Salzburg consensus criteria for non-convulsive status epilepticus: Approach to clinical application. Epilepsy & Behavior. 2015;**49**:158-163

[26] Leitinger M, Trinka E, Gardella E, Rohracher A, Kalss G, Qerama E, et al. Diagnostic accuracy of the Salzburg EEG criteria for non-convulsive status epilepticus: A retrospective study. Lancet Neurology. 2016;**15**:1054-1062

[27] Mesraoua B, Deleu D, Hail Al H. et al. Nonconvulsive Status Epilepticus in Patients with Altered Mental Status Admitted to Hamad. DOI: 10.5772/intechopen.83580

[28] Trinka E, Cock H, Hesdor er D, et al. A definition and classication of status epilepticus—Report of the ILAE task force on classification of status epilepticus. Epilepsia. 2015;**56**:1515-1523

[29] Naravanan JT, Murthy JM. Nonconvulsive status epilepticus in a neurological intensive care unit: Profile in a developing country. Epilepsy. 2007;**5**:900-906

[30] Young GB, Jordan KG, Doig GS. An assessment of nonconvulsive seizures in the intensive care unit using continuous EEG monitoring: An investigation of variables associated with mortality. Neurology. 1996;**47**(1):83-89

[31] Litt B, Wityk RJ, Hertz SH, Mullen PD, Weiss H, Ryan DD, et al. Nonconvulsive status epilepticus in the critically ill elderly. Epilepsia. 1998;**39**(11):1194-1202

[32] Trinka E, Leitinger M. Which EEG patterns in coma are nonconvulsive status epilepticus? Epilepsy & Behavior. 2015;**49**:203-222

[33] Baykal B, Ebru A, editors. Nonconvulsive Status Epilepticus. Istanbul: Cortex Publishing; 2018

Chapter 4

Meningococcal Meningitis

Trond Flægstad

Abstract

Meningococcal disease may present as meningitis, septicemia, or a combination of the two. Generally, meningitis has a gradual onset, with fever, headache, and neck stiffness as the most frequent clinical symptoms. By contrast, fulminant septicemia may develop within hours, and is characterized by petechial bleedings and shock. It is of vital importance to diagnose and treat meningococcal disease rapidly. The diagnosis is based on the culture of Neisseria meningitides from blood or cerebrospinal fluid, or on the polymerase chain reaction (PCR) of spinal fluid. Cefotaxime or ceftriaxone are usually recommended as antibacterial treatment. There is a vaccine effective against disease with serogroups A, C, Y, and W.

Keywords: meningococci, meningitis, Neisseria, vaccine

1. Clinical features of meningococcal disease

Meningococcal disease is one of the most devastating infections in an individual or community, and is caused by the bacterium *Neisseria meningitidis* with diseases most often in the forms of meningitis, septicemia, or a combination of meningitis and septicemia [1–4]. The onset can be nonspecific, but is usually abrupt with symptoms as fever, malaise, and myalgia, and a rash that initially may be urticarial, maculopapular, or petechial (purpuric). Fulminant meningococcal septicemia is usually characterized by the rapid development of hypotension, ecchymosis, and disseminated intravascular coagulation (DIC).

Meningitis is characterized by gradual onset of fever, headache, neck-stiffness, backache, and nausea.

In meningococcal meningitis, drowsiness, reduced cognitive function, stiff neck, and positive Kernig and Brudzinski's signs, all manifestations of meningeal inflammation, are usually present along with fever. Neurological findings may be cranial nerve dysfunction, seizures, focal cerebral signs, and reduced consciousness. The symptoms and signs of meningococcal meningitis are indistinguishable from those associated with acute meningitis caused by *Haemophilus influenzae* type b bacteria, *Streptococcus pneumoniae*, and other bacteria. However, the presence of petechiae strongly implicates *N. meningitidis.*

2. Typing systems and classification of *Neisseria meningitidis*

N. meningitidis is a Gram-negative diplococcus. Several methods for typing and classification of *N. meningitidis* exist. The system currently used most widely is based on antigenic differences of different bacterial surface structures and on susceptibility to sulfonamides. According to this scheme, meningococci are classified by:

(a) serogroup (capsular polysaccharides) (A, B, C, X, Y, W are most common in invasive disease); (b) serotype (the class 2 or 3 outer-membrane proteins); and (c) subtype (the class 1 outer-membrane protein). The phenotype of a meningococcus is written: serogroup:serotype:subtype. According to this, the epidemic strain in North Norway (serogroup B, serotype 15, subtype P1.7.16) is designated: B:15:P1.7.16 [5].

3. Epidemiology of meningococcal meningitis

N. meningitidis only infects humans; there is no animal reservoir. The bacteria can be carried in the throat and sometimes, for reasons not fully understood, can overwhelm the body's defenses allowing infection to spread through the bloodstream to the brain. It is believed that 1–10% of the population carries *N. meningitidis* in their throat at any given time. However, the carriage rate may be higher in epidemic situations [6].

The bacteria are transmitted from person to person through droplets of respiratory or throat secretions from carriers. Close and prolonged contact—such as kissing, sneezing or coughing on someone, or living in close quarters (such as a dormitory, sharing eating or drinking utensils) with an infected person facilitates the spread of the disease. The average incubation period is 4 days, but can range between 2 and 10 days.

Meningococcal disease occurs in almost every country in the world regardless of climate and economic development. Serogroup A disease has been most often associated with widespread epidemics in Africa where epidemics of serogroup A meningococcal disease tends to occur every 7–10 years in sub-Saharan Africa (**Figure 1**).

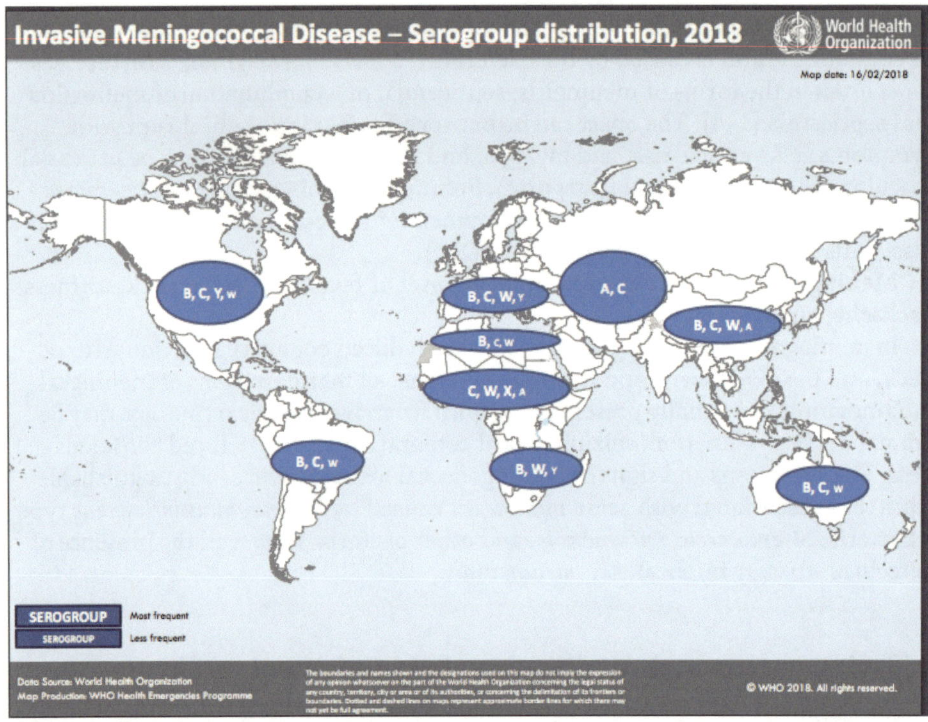

Figure 1.
Serogroup distribution of invasive meningococcal disease, 2018. Source: http://www.who.int/emergencies/diseases/meningitis/serogroup-distribution-2018.pdf.

The highest rate of meningococcal disease occurs in children below 4 years of age, but all age groups may be affected [5–7].

The overall mortality rate for invasive meningococcal disease is 10–15%, while about 15% of the survivors suffer from permanent sequelae like hearing impairment, neurological disability, and digit or limb amputation [3].

In 2015, there were 379,000 deaths caused by meningitis worldwide, of those 73,000 by *N. meningitis*; most of these deaths were in children less than 5 years of age [6, 8].

4. Laboratory diagnosis of meningococcal meningitis

Initially, the diagnosis of meningococcal disease rests on clinical signs and symptoms. On admission, appropriate specimens should be immediately collected to ensure correct diagnosis.

4.1 Collection of appropriate specimens for bacteriological analysis

Antibacterial treatment of suspected meningococcal meningitis must be started as soon as possible and is often initiated before admission. To ensure correct diagnosis, it is important to collect bacteriological specimens before therapy is started. At the hospital, blood culture should always be collected. Cerebrospinal fluid (CSF) is collected for microscopy, culture, and detection of meningococci by antigen testing or by polymerase chain reaction (PCR). One drop of CSF is collected on microscope slide and dried in air for microscopy. One or two drops of CSF are tapped on a swab and placed in a tube of Amies or Stuart transport medium for culture. When placed in a transport medium, the bacteria will stay alive for a longer period of time than in liquid.

CSF can also be collected in a liquid culture medium, like a blood culture medium. Some laboratories supply clinical departments with agar culture media so that CSF can be collected directly on them before being sent to the laboratory. Finally, 1 ml of liquid CSF is collected in a sterile container for bacterial culture and polymerase chain reaction (PCR).

Because meningococci survive longer in the throat than in the CSF and blood after antibacterial treatment has started, a throat sample is highly recommended. The specimens should be sent to the laboratory and processed immediately. If the specimens have to be stored before transport, they should preferably be kept at 8–10°C or at room temperature. Petechial skin lesions also represent a potential diagnostic specimen. Meningococci are often present in the petechiae, and Gram-stain smears and culture of needle aspirates or punch biopsies from skin lesions are positive in up to 60% of cases [9]. This can be particularly useful when antibiotic treatment was started before cultures were obtained.

PCR can detect small quantities of bacterial DNA and is useful, because of results may be obtained after a few hours, and sensitivity is not affected by previous antibiotic treatment [10].

4.2 Microbiological diagnosis of meningococcal meningitis

4.2.1 Culture

Conventionally, culture is the standard method for making a diagnosis of meningococcal disease. If the specimens have to be stored before transport, they should preferably be kept at 4°C for CSF in order to be analyzed by PCR or at room temperature (suitable for the strains in Amies medium, or cultures on chocolate agar medium) in order to be analyzed.

In the microbiology laboratory, CSF from patients with suspected meningococcal meningitis is cultured on blood agar and chocolate agar overnight at 36.5–37.0°C in 10% CO_2. In some laboratories, CSF is also cultured in blood-culture bottles or in another liquid medium. Throat specimens are cultured on agar media selecting growth of meningococci. Blood is cultured in commercially available bottles containing a rich culture medium supporting the growth of a wide range of bacteria.

4.2.2 Microscopy and agglutination methods

A Gram-stained preparat of CSF is most often analyzed. Meningococci typically are seen as Gram-negative [red] coffee bean-like diplococci. A fluorescent staining method using acridine-orange which stains bacteria orange-red and human cells pale yellow has also proved valuable. Agglutination method, directly from sediment coming from CSF, after centrifugation, can be used to determine meningococcal serogroup, except for serogroup B.

4.2.3 Genetic methods

Microbial nucleic acids are stable and can be detected in body fluids and tissues even though the microbes are dead and are in very small quantities. Real-time PCR can give results in approximately 2 h, much easier by comparing with conventional PCR, and can give species and serogroup identification.

4.3 Nonbacterial tests

In meningococcal meningitis, the number of leukocytes and levels of acute phase proteins such as procalcitonin and C-reactive protein in the blood are normally elevated. The number of leukocytes in CSF usually exceeds 800 cells/mm^3, and there is a relative increase in the number of granulocytes. The concentration of protein is increased and that of sugar decreased. In early stages of meningococcal meningitis, leukocytes may be absent from the CSF, although the culture later may grow meningococci. The absence of leucocytes does therefore not exclude bacterial meningitis.

5. Treatment of meningococcal meningitis

5.1 General principles

National and international guidelines for treatment of meningococcal disease exist, and our recommendations are based generally on these guidelines [3, 11]. In addition to prompt use of antimicrobial agents, the immediate treatment of increased intracranial pressure, seizures, and shock if present, must be started, and normal hydration and electrolyte balance must be restored. Because shock is a very early event and can often be life threatening, its management should take precedence over fluid restrictions aimed at preventing the inappropriate secretion of antidiuretic hormone. Infants with vomiting may show relative hypovolemia.

There is no report supporting the use of prophylactic glucocorticoid therapy in meningococcal meningitis. The majority of patients enrolled in trials with adjunctive dexamethasone therapy are children with *H. influenzae* meningitis. The benefits of glucocorticoid therapy may not extend to children with other pathogens, and the benefit in adults is even less clear.

5.2 Principles of antimicrobial treatment

Bacterial meningitis is an infection in an area of impaired host resistance. Specific antibodies and complement are frequently absent from the cerebrospinal fluid in patients with meningococcal meningitis, resulting in inefficient phagocytosis and subsequent rapid bacterial multiplication. It is therefore necessary to treat meningitis with antimicrobial agents that are bactericidal, penetrate to the CSF easily, and rapidly reach bactericidal concentrations. The increased permeability of the blood-brain barrier during meningeal infection enhances the penetration of most antibiotics into CSF.

In experimental meningitis, it has been found that maximal bactericidal activity of an antibacterial agent occurs at a concentration 10–30 times greater than the minimal in vitro bactericidal concentration. Cranial imaging is required before spinal puncture in patients who are in coma, have papilledema, or have focal neurological symptoms. Before imaging, adequate clinical specimens must be collected and empirical therapy started. Empirical therapy must be selected on the basis of the age of the patient, symptoms, and the local frequency of etiological bacterial pathogens.

In cases of suspected bacterial meningitis (or meningococcal sepsis), patients should be treated empirically to cover the most likely pathogens while awaiting culture results. Cefotaxime or ceftriaxone is usually recommended [3]. This might be changed to penicillin G when the diagnosis is bacteriologically confirmed. For patients with a life-threatening penicillin allergy characterized by anaphylaxis, chloramphenicol is recommended.

The duration of therapy is normally 7 days. Rare isolates of beta-lactamase producing meningococcal strains with high-level resistance have been described, as have clinical isolates with altered penicillin-binding proteins and intermediate resistance to penicillin [MIC, 0.1–1.0 g/l]. Since many of these patients were successfully treated with benzylpenicillin, the importance of in vitro penicillin insensitivity in meningococci is unclear.

6. Prevention of meningococcal meningitis

6.1 Primary prevention of meningococcal disease

Vaccines against meningococcal disease exist, but protection is only against meningococcal disease of the same capsular polysaccharide present in the vaccine. A present, there are vaccines against serogroups A, C, Y, and W; commonly combined in a quadrivalent conjugated vaccine (A, C, Y, W).

Recommended immunization with this vaccine is for children and adults with complement deficiency, asplenia, who are at risk during a community outbreak attributable to a vaccine serogroup, are residents or will travel to endemic areas, or are HIV positive [3]. The conjugate vaccines confer long-lasting immunity (5 years or more), prevent carriage, and induce herd immunity.

Polysaccharide vaccines are used during a response to outbreaks, mainly in Africa. They are either bivalent (A, C); trivalent (A, C, W); or tetravalent (A, C, Y, W) [6]. They are not effective before 2 years of age, offer a 3-year protection but do not induce herd immunity.

At present, there is no long-lasting protective vaccine against the serogroup B meningococcus, but it is used in outbreak response [6].

6.2 Secondary prevention of meningococcal disease

Following a case of meningococcal disease, contacts should be vaccinated if the causative strain belongs to a serogroup against which a protective vaccine exists (A, C, Y, and W). However, it takes 2–3 weeks to produce protective antibodies, during which period secondary disease may develop. The use of chemoprophylaxis to eradicate the disease-causing strain from close contact, thereby stopping the spread of the infection, is therefore recommended. Household members of a patient with meningococcal disease have a much higher risk of contracting the disease than the general population. Household members of the patient and kissing contacts are most likely to carry the disease-causing strain and need chemoprophylaxis. Other close contacts to whom chemoprophylaxis may be considered are babysitters including grandparents or other family members, and kindergarten employees. Rifampicin, ceftriaxone, or ciprofloxacin are the recommended drugs [3].

Acknowledgements

The publication charges for this article have been funded by a grant from the publication fund of UiT The Arctic University of Norway.

Author details

Trond Flægstad
University and University Hospital of Tromsø, Norway

*Address all correspondence to: trond.flaegstad@unn.no

References

[1] Stephens DSGB, Brandtzaeg P. Epidemic meningitis, meningococcaemia, and Neisseria meningitidis. Lancet. 2007;**369**(9580):2196-2210

[2] Viner RM, Booy R, Johnson H, Edmunds WJ, Hudson L, Bedford H, et al. Outcomes of invasive meningococcal serogroup B disease in children and adolescents (MOSAIC): A case-control study. The Lancet Neurology. 2012;**11**(9):774-783

[3] Kimberlin DW, Brady MT, Jackson MA, editors. Red book: Report form the Committee on Infectious Diseases, Meningococcal Infections. 31 ed. Elk Grove Village, Ill., USA: American Academy of Pediatrics; 2018

[4] Kristiansen BE, Flægstad T. Guidelines for the diagnosis and treatment of meningococcal meningitis. Disease Management & Health Outcomes. 1999;**5**(2):73-81

[5] Nordheim K, Hovland IH, Kristiansen BE, Kaaresen PI, Flaegstad T. An epidemic of meningococcal disease in children in North Norway in the 1970s and 1980s was dominated by a hypervirulent group B strain. Acta Paediatrica. 2018;**107**(3):490-495

[6] Meningococcal meningitis: WHO. 2018. Available from: http://www.who.int/en/news-room/fact-sheets/detail/meningococcal-meningitis

[7] MacNeil JR, Blain AE, Wang X, Cohn AC. Current Epidemiology and trends in meningococcal disease-United States, 1996-2015. Clinical Infectious Diseases: An Official Publication of the Infectious Diseases Society of America. 2018;**66**(8):1276-1281

[8] Mortality GBD, Causes of Death C. Global, regional, and national life expectancy, all-cause mortality, and cause-specific mortality for 249 causes of death, 1980-2015: A systematic analysis for the Global Burden of Disease Study 2015. Lancet. 2016;**388**(10053):1459-1544

[9] Arend SM, Lavrijsen AP, Kuijken I, van der Plas RN, Kuijper EJ. Prospective controlled study of the diagnostic value of skin biopsy in patients with presumed meningococcal disease. European journal of clinical microbiology & infectious diseases: Official publication of the European Society of Clinical. Microbiology. 2006;**25**(10):643-649

[10] Bryant PA, Li HY, Zaia A, Griffith J, Hogg G, Curtis N, et al. Prospective study of a real-time PCR that is highly sensitive, specific, and clinically useful for diagnosis of meningococcal disease in children. Journal of Clinical Microbiology. 2004;**42**(7):2919-2925

[11] Defeating bacterial meningitis: WHO; 2018. Available from: http://www.who.int/emergencies/diseases/meningitis/en/

Chapter 5

Healthcare-Associated Meningitis Caused by *M. tuberculosis* and Non-Tuberculous Mycobacteria

Ashit Bhusan Xess, Kiran Bala and Urvashi B. Singh

Abstract

Meningitis can be acquired in the community setting or secondary to invasive procedures or head trauma. The latter group has been classified as health-care-associated meningitis because the etiologic agents belong to a different spectrum of microorganisms, including *Staphylococcus aureus*, Coagulase negative staphylococcus Gram negative bacilli, Aspergillus, *Candida albicans*, *Cryptococcus neoformans*. IDSA Clinical Practice guidelines for Healthcare-associated ventriculitis and meningitis does not include *M. tuberculosis* and NTM, but in the last decade infections caused by these organisms are on a rise. These infections are mostly associated with cerebrospinal fluid shunts, cerebrospinal fluid drains, intra-thecal drug therapy, deep brain stimulation hardware, neurosurgery and head trauma. Most commonly these are introduced during surgical procedures. Another important pathogenic factor is biofilm formation that increases the persistence and resistance to antibiotic therapy, hence the survival. A high index of suspicion aids early diagnosis but preventive measures such as care of the devices introduced into sterile spaces is essential. Sterilization of the critical items is recommended by treating with different chemical sterilizing agents but most importantly meticulous cleaning must precede any high-level disinfection or sterilization process. A course of multidrug therapy is required for prolonged period of time depending on mycobacterial species.

Keywords: non-tuberculous mycobacteria, *Mycobacterium tuberculosis*, hospital acquired infections, iatrogenic infections

1. Introduction

Healthcare-associated CNS infection mostly includes meningitis, ventriculitis, subdural empyema and brain abscess. With increased use of intracranial devices and increase in number of patients requiring neurosurgery, the risk of acquiring these infections has increased. While these devices generally being sterile, they can provide a route for microorganism during placement, handling or maintenance. The most common causative agents are Staphylococcus aureus, coagulase negative staphylococcus, Gram-negative bacteria, candida species, Cryptococcus neoformans, etc. In the last decade, Mycobacterium tuberculosis and non-tuberculous mycobacterium are gaining prominence in causing healthcare-associated CNS infections. These organisms especially non-tuberculous mycobacterium are found in environment which once find entry into CNS can cause infections. No approved treatment guidelines are present for the treatment of non-tuberculous mycobacterium. So one must take utmost care in maintaining these intracranial devices from not acquiring these infections. These devices and neurosurgical devices come under critical category as per Spaulding classification, so stringent decontamination and sterilization procedures have to be followed to render them sterile.

2. Meningitis

Meningitis is an acute inflammation of the protective membranes covering the brain and spinal cord known collectively as the meninges which consists of duramater, arachnoid mater and pia mater [1].

The patient with meningitis usually presents with fever, headache, altered sensorium, behavioral changes, focal neurological signs or seizures. There are various signs that can be elicited in meningitis patients such as nuchal rigidity, Kernig's sign and Brudzinski's sign. Nuchal rigidity or neck rigidity is elicited when neck resists passive flexion. Kernig's sign is elicited on a supine position where knees are flexed onto the abdomen. Any attempt to extend the knee from this position causes pain in the patient. Brudzinski's sign is also elicited in supine position where trying to flex the neck causes flexion at the knee and hip joints. These signs indicate there is meningeal irritation in the patient. But both these tests are uncertain in some cases such as in very young or old patients, immunocompromised or patients with depressed mental status.

Meningitis can be divided into acute, subacute and chronic meningitis. Acute meningitis is mostly caused by bacteria whereas subacute and chronic also include viral, fungal and parasitic causes. In cases of acute meningitis most common causes are Neisseria meningitides, *Streptococcus pneumoniae*, *Escherichia coli*, *Pseudomonas aeruginosa*, Staphylococcus species, *Listeria monocytogenes*, *Haemophilus influenzae*, *Streptococcus agalactiae*, *Bacteroides fragilis* and *Fusobacterium* species. Viral causes include Enteroviruses, Herpes Zoster virus, Herpes Simplex viruse 2, Epstein Barr virus, Human Immunodeficiency virus (**Table 1**).

Organisms causing subacute meningitis consists of *Mycobacterium tuberculosis*, *Cryptococcus neoformans*, *Histoplasma capsulatum*, *Coccidioides immitis* and *Treponema pallidum*. Bacterial agents causing chronic meningitis are *Mycobacterium tuberculosis*, *Borrelia burgdorferi* and *Treponema pallidum*. Fungal agents comprises of *Cryptococcus neoformans*, *Coccidiodes immitis*, *Candida* species, *Histoplasma capsulatum*, *Blastomyces dermatitidis*, *Aspergillus* species and *Sporothrix schenckii*. Helminthic causes are *Taenia solium*, *Gnathostoma spinigerum*, *Angiostrongylus cantonensis* [2].

2.1 Healthcare-associated meningitis

Meningitis can be acquired in community settings or in hospital settings via invasive procedures performed or through head trauma. In hospital settings the causative agents are totally different from those acquired in community settings. In many of the cases the symptoms appear after discharge from the hospital. There are many ways in which a patient can acquire meningitis in a hospital settings which are as follows [3]:

- CSF shunts
- CSF drains
- Intrathecal infusion pumps
- Deep brain stimulation hardware
- Neurosurgery

ACUTE MENINGITIS	SUBACUTE MENINGITIS	CHRONIC MENINGITIS
Neisseria meningitides	Mycobacterium tuberculosis	Mycobacterium tuberculosis
Streptococcus pneumonia	Treponema pallidum	Borrelia burgdorferi
Escherichia coli	**Fungal causes**	Treponema pallidum
Pseudomonas aeruginosa	Cryptococcus neoformans	**Fungal causes**
Staphylococcus species	Histoplasma capsulatum	Cryptococcus neoformans
Listeria monoocytogenes	Coccidioides immitis	Coccidioides immitis
Haemophilus influenzae		Candida species
Streptococcus agalactiae		Histoplasma capsulatum
Bacteroides fragilis		Blastomyces dermatitidis
Fusobacterim species		Aspergillus species
Viral causes		Sporothrix schenkii
Enteroviruses		**Helminthic causes**
Herpes zoster virus		Taenia solium
Herpes simplex virus 2		Gnathostoma spinigerum
Epstein barr virus		Angiostrongylus cantonensis
Human immunodeficiency virus		

Table 1.
Causative agents of meningitis.

2.1.1 Cereberospinal fluid shunts

CSF shunt is a system in which the proximal part of it is in the cerebral ventricle, subdural space, intracranial cyst or lumbar arachnoid space whereas the distal end is in the peritoneal, pleural or vascular space. A part of the system has a pressure regulating valve which usually is present just outside the skull or in the distal part of the system. Additional connecting systems may be present which facilitates connection of more catheters or devices [4].

The incidence of CSF shunt infections may show huge variations in various studies but it usually ranges from 4 to 17% [5, 6]. Factors associated with CSF shunt infections can be divided into preoperative and operative causes. Preoperative causes includes premature birth associated with intraventricular hemorrhage, younger age, previous shunt infections, hydrocephalus caused by purulent meningitis, hemorrhage or myelomeningocele. Operative causes are inexperienced neurosurgeon, movement of people during procedure, perforated surgical gloves, neuroendoscope use, longer duration of procedure, insertion of catheter below T7 vertebral body in case of ventriculoarterial shunting, improper patient skin preparation, shaving of skin, large areas of skin exposed during procedure and repeated shunt revision surgeries [7, 8].

There are 4 possible mechanisms by which CSF shunts can get infected. First and most frequent mechanism is colonization of the shunt during surgery. The second mechanism is retrograde infection from the distal end of the shunt. This can be due to bowel perforation or surgeries being conducted in gastrointestinal tract or genitourinary tract. Due to the breach in the GI tract there is a possibility of retrograde infections by microbial flora of GI tract. Third mechanism is through skin after injection of drug into ventricular reservoir or assess potency. Fourth mechanism is through haematogenous seeding in cases of ventriculoarterial shunts wherein bacteremia is the cause of retrograde infections [3].

2.1.2 Cerebrospinal fluid drains

CSF drains are temporary catheters used to divert CSF externally into a collecting bag. These are used in the temporary management of elevated intracranial pressure due to acute hydrocephalus secondary to intracranial hemorrhage, neoplasm, obstruction of the CSF circulation or trauma. The proximal end of the catheter is usually situated in the cerebral ventricle, subdural space, intracranial cyst or lumbar subarachnoid space. The distal end is connected to a collecting system which consists of a drip chamber, ports for measuring intracranial pressure, ports for sampling and collecting bag. Studies have shown the incidence rates may range from 0 to 22%. In a study by Ramanan et al., the overall external ventricular drain related infection was found to be 11.4 per 1000 catheter days [9].

Factors associated with increased risk of infections in external CSF drains are intraventricular or subarachnoid hemorrhage, cranial fracture with CSF leak, catheter irrigation, craniotomy and duration of catheterization. Mechanisms generally include introduction of microorganism during the procedure, by retrograde infections through exit ports and during flushing of the tubings to maintain patency [3].

2.1.3 Intrathecal infusion pumps

Intrathecal infusion pumps are used as drug delivery systems in conditions such as cerebral palsy, multiple sclerosis, trauma, hereditary spastic paraplegia to deliver baclofen in order to relieve the spasticity. Through these delivery systems opiates are administered in management of intractable pain usually in cases of malignancy. The catheter of these pumps are inserted at the lumbar region and passed intrathecally to the point where drug has to be delivered. Generally these pumps are placed subcutaneously in the abdomen region but in pediatric patients these devices are placed under the abdominal fascia. These pumps have to be refilled from time to time transcutaneously with the desired drug [3].

Majority of the cases who get infected or contract meningitis consists of pediatric patients [10, 11]. Majority of the infections occur within 2 months of surgery but it can happen anytime in the next 3–6 months where drug is refilling is being done. Infection rates may vary from 3.6% in subfacially placed pumps to 20% in subcutaneously placed pumps [12]. In many studies it is seen that it is difficult to distinguish meningitis from local infections. In a study out of 207 children with infusion pumps 25 had suspected superficial infections, 13 had deep seated infections and only 2 of them had meningitis [13]. Route of entry for these infections are during surgery or during refilling of the pumps.

2.1.4 Deep brain stimulation hardware

Deep brain stimulation is used in cases of parkinsonism, dystonia, essential tremors and obsessive-compulsive disorders. This whole set up consists of intracranial lead, connector and a pulse generator implanted in infraclavicular area. In cases of intractable focal epilepsy cortical and depth electrodes are placed which not only detects abnormal electroencephalographic activity but also delivers patterned electrical stimuli to interrupt seizures.

The infections can occur during initial surgery or following surgery performed in order to replace the battery. The infection of pulse generator is the most common infection. There might be a retrograde infection from the pulse generator which can cause meningitis. The incidence of infection may vary from 0.62 to 14.3% and may involve all the 3 components of the device [14].

2.1.5 Neurosurgery

In cases of neurosurgery there is higher risk of ventriculitis and meningitis since there is direct manipulation of central nervous system. So the infections can be introduced during surgical procedure through various instruments or even surgeons themselves. The instruments may be at fault if they are not sterilized. Surgeons on the other hand if are not following proper hand washing practices might be the source of infection. In a study conducted in Taiwan the incidence of bacterial meningitis in a tertiary care hospital was 48% [15].

According to 2017 IDSA Clinical Practice Guidelines for Healthcare-Associated Ventriculitis and Meningitis all the above organisms mentioned in **Table 2** are common agents of healthcare-associated meningitis. *Mycobacterium tuberculosis* and non-tuberculous mycobacterium does not find mention in the above list. But there are adequate number of cases wherein *Mycobacterium* species especially non-tuberculous mycobacterium are causative agents of nosocomial meningitis.

2.2 *Mycobacterium tuberculosis* and non-tuberculous mycobacterium (NTM)

Traditionally *Mycobacterium* species has been classified according to phenotypic characteristics (**Table 3**) but with the advent of molecular studies characterization

Gram Positive Agents	Gram Negative Agents	Fungal Agents
• Coagulase Negative Staphylococcus (e.g. Staphylococcus epidermidis) • Staphylococcus aureus • Propionibacterium acnes	• Escherichia coli • Enterobacter species • Citrobacter species • Serratia species • Pseudomonas aeruginosa • Acinetobacter species	• Candida species • Exserohilum species

Table 2.
Causative agents of healthcare acquired meningitis.

Mycobacterium tuberculosis Complex	Nontuberculous Mycobacteria			
	Photochromogens	Nonphotochromogens	Scotochromogens	Rapid Growers
M.tuberculosis	M.kansasii	M.avium complex	M.schulzai	M.fortuitum
M.bovis	M.asiaticum	M.intercellulare	M.scrofulaeceum	M.chelonae
M.bovis BCG	M.marinum	M.ulcerans	M.interjectum	M.abscessus
M.africanum		M.celatum	M.gordonae	M.smegmatis
M.caprae		M.gastri	M.cookii	M.peregrinum
M.canetti		M.genavense	M.hiberniae	M.immunogenum
M.microti		M.haemophilum	M.lentiflavum	M.goodii
M.pinnepedii		M.malmoense	M.conspicuum	M.septicum
		M.shimoidei	M.heckeshornense	M. houstonense
		M.xenopi	M.tusciae	M.mucogenicum
		M.heidelbergense	M.kubicae	M.neworleansense
		M.branderi	M.ulcerans	M.brisbanense
		M.simiae	M.bohemicum	M.senegalense
		M.triplex		
		M.conspicuum		

Table 3.
Classification of genus Mycobacterium.

of these organisms are done at genetic level. The organisms belonging to genus *Mycobacterium* are aerobic, non-spore forming, non-motile, thin, slightly curved or straight rods. *Mycobacterium* species have a cell wall comprising of N-glycolylmuramic acid which has a very high lipid content. Because of this property it creates a hydrophobic permeability barrier. The growth rate of these organisms is very slow because of their hydrophobic cell surface. Because of the hydrophobicity these organisms tend to clump with each other which results in reduced diffusion of nutrients into the cell. The generation time for mycobacterium is about 20–36 h [16].

2.3 *Mycobacterium tuberculosis* and healthcare-associated infections

M. tuberculosis is the major cause of infectious health burden in the whole world. In the developing countries tuberculosis is a major concern in the population. Tuberculosis not only involves the respiratory system but also every system in the body. This is why tuberculosis is not only a health burden but also a social burden and economic burden on any nation.

M. tuberculosis becomes more lethal because of its latency. It is capable of going into a phase of latency wherein there are no symptoms at all to suggest the patient is infected. When the patients' immune system weakens these organisms find an opportunity to reactivate and affect any organ system in the body. Patients who come for different conditions to the hospital have weakened immune system. So it might so happen that these organisms may reactivate and affect the patient.

A study has shown that *M. tuberculosis* has been majorly involved in prosthetic joint infections [17]. In this study 53% of the cases were hip joint infections, 40.9% cases involved knee joint and rest were other joints. One reason could be that in patients with latent infections the infected monocytes migrate towards sites of inflammation i.e. surgical sites and cause prosthetic joint infections [18, 19]. Another reason could be that surgical trauma could break down old granulomas and hence reactivation of tuberculosis in the joints [20, 21].

Another site that *M. tuberculosis* is known to infect is the pacemaker implantation site. In a study by Al-Ghamdi it was found out of 25 cases of pacemaker implantation site infection 8 cases comprised of *M. tuberculosis* infection and others were NTM [22]. These sites were infected via haematogenous route.

2.4 Non-tuberculous mycobacteria and healthcare acquired infections

The NTM group consists of more than 172 different species implicated in different clinical conditions (http://www.bacterionet/mycobacterium.html). NTM are important environmental opportunistic pathogens of humans and animals including poultry and fish. The NTM are ubiquitous in nature and are found in various habitats. In the past few years NTM are isolated from natural sources like water, soil, animals, milk, food products and from artificial resources such as water distribution systems and sewer [23, 24].

Unlike *Mycobacterium tuberculosis*, notification of NTM is not mandatory because of which accurate knowledge of impact of NTM on public health is unknown. The impact of NTM is significantly seen in immunocompromised patients e.g. AIDS and transplant patients as life-threatening opportunistic infections [25, 26]. Off late there has been a surge in pulmonary infections and hospital acquired infections (HAI) in immunocompetent patients suggesting the importance of NTM on human health [27–30]. NTMs are implicated in medical device related infections because of their biofilm capabilities [31]. Their ubiquitous nature allows them to cause persistent infection in the patients in healthcare settings [32].

2.4.1 Non-tuberculous mycobacterium and biofilms

In the early days of Mycobacteriology Lowenstein and Calmette described the phenomenon of mycobacterial cells forming aggregates and pellicles [33, 34], whereas Robert Koch described these cells pressed together and arranged in bundles [35]. These were the earlier days when we see description which are similar to the picture of biofilm formation in the present day. The first report of modern concept of biofilms was published by costerton [36]. A decade later articles began to appear about environmental mycobacterial biofilms [37, 38].

Biofilm formation by mycobacteria are no different from the process by which other bacteria form biofilms. It starts with bacterial adhesion goes through stages of surface attachment, sessile growth, matrix synthesis and dispersion. Intercellular communication happens through quorum sensing [39]. However mycobacterial biofilms can form on air-liquid interface. This happens because of composition of extracellular matrix. The extracellular matrix consists of short mycolic acid which are hydrophobic in nature and because of this property biofilms are formed at the air-media interface [40]. In a study it has been shown maximum thickness for *M. fortuitum* and *M. chelonae* biofilm was detected by 72 h but other non-pigmented RGM reach maximum thickness by 96 h. *M. chelonae* covers smaller surface area than *M. abscessus*, but greater area than *M. fortuitum* and *M. margeritense*. *M. chelonae* forms a biofilm which grows vertically whereas *M. fortuitum* covers the entire surface with thinner growth. Extensive cording is seen in *M. abscessus* and *M. chelonae* [41].

NTM are considered as etiological agents of healthcare-associated infections (HAI), which is a major public health concern. These are responsible for colonization of respiratory tract, infections related to medical procedures and disseminated infections in immunocompromised. Earlier *M. avium* used to be the main cause but RGMs like *M. fortuitum*, *M. abscessus* and *M. chelonae* are growing into prominence [42–44]. The main reason is biofilm formation by NTM. NTM organized in biofilms are hard to eradicate by common disinfection process and disinfectants such as chlorine, organomercurials, alkaline glutaraldehydes [43, 45–47]. Biofilms are also highly resistant to antimicrobial drugs and are able to modulate the host immune response [48]. This is due to physical barrier formed by the biofilm itself and also due to horizontal gene transfer between cells [49]. Bacteria also can switch their phenotypic stages causing a slower growth rate hence the effect of drugs acting on replicating organisms is nullified. These bacteria are known as persisters [50].

It has been proved in studies that NTM form biofilms on medical devices which in turn causes persistent infections. In a study it has been shown NTM form biofilms on silicone which are used to coat medical devices e.g. endoscopes, catheters and air-liquid interface. Biofilms formed by *M. fortuitum* and *M. abscessus* have higher bacterial load than *M. chelonae*. *M. fortuitum* is considered as a good biofilm assembler [51].

2.5 Non-tuberculous mycobacteria and healthcare-associated meningitis

In the review of spectrum of CNS disease caused by RGM by Talati et al., [52] 19 cases of primary and secondary CNS infections were reported, fourteen cases were caused by *M. fortuitum*. Most common clinical presentation in the study was subacute meningitis, with symptom duration ranging from 3 days to 5 months. There are other isolated reports, where *Mycobacterium fortuitum* is the cause of CNS infections. **Table 4** summarizes cases isolated from CNS after VP shunt insertion. There are two other reported cases of VP shunt infection due to *M. abscessus*, a 30 yr. old male with hydrocephalus [53] and a 59-year-old man with hydrocephalus [54] (reported by us previously). Post insertion of VP shunt, the patients presented with meningeal signs and symptoms; but time duration for onset of symptoms varied from 8 days to months and in two cases, 16 and 30 years [55–58]. Other reports of cases of CNS infections due to *M. fortuitum* associated with intra-thecal pump infections, epidural catheter, balloon mitral valvotomy, chronic suppurative otitis media, mastoiditis, sacral trauma, meningioma resection have been published [59–61]. Literature reveals, only 6 cases of VP shunt due to *M. fortuitum* and *M. abscessus* (4, 2 cases respectively), causing CNS infections worldwide.

A 14 year old girl with high grade fever and altered sensorium was received in the emergency department of our institution. She had a past history of persistent headache and seizures. CT scan revealed posterior fossa glioma but could not be operated on since it was very near to the vital parts of the brain. So V-P shunt was placed in order to relieve the ventricular obstruction. After 3 years she underwent appendicectomy after which she started to have frequent convulsions. CT scan revealed dilated ventricles for which a revision shunt surgery was performed. But the symptoms were not relieved. Therefore shunt surgeries were performed without any improvement in the symptoms. In our institution we received the csf sample

S. no.	Authors	Country	Age/Sex	Underlying disease	Mode of acquisition	Mycobacterial spp	Treatment	Duration of therapy	Outcome
1.	Chan et al (1991) [57]	Hong Kong	60yr/F	Cerebral haemorrhage	V-A shunt	M. fortuitum	IV amikacin, ofloxacin	2.5 months	Alive
2.	Midani et al (1999) [56]	USA	13yr/ F	Spina bifida	V-P shunt	M. fortuitum	IV amikacin, cotrimoxazole	7.5 months	Alive
3.	Vishwanathan et al (2004) [58]	India	60 yrs/M	Traumatic Brain injury	Ventriculo arterial shunt	M. fortuitum	IV Kanamycin, ciprofloxacin	6 months	Alive
4.	Cadena et al (2014) [55]	USA	14 yrs/M	Congenital hydrocephalus	V-P shunt	M. fortuitum	IV meropenem, oral cotrimoxazole, oral moxifloxacin		Alive
5.	Baidya A, Singh U B (2016) [54]	India	59yrs/M	Tubercular Meningitis/ hydrocephalus	V-P shunt	M. abscessus	IV amikacin, clarithromycin, meropenem Shunt removal	One week	Died
6.	Montero et al (2016) [53]	USA	30yrs/M	Hydrocephalus	V-P shunt	M. abscessus	IV Azithromycin, Imipenem,amikacin Shunt removal	Two years	Alive
7.	Present case	India	14yrs/F	Glioma/ Hydrocephalus	V-P shunt	M. fortuitum	IV Linezolid, ofloxacin, clofazimine, clarithromycin.	continuing	Alive

Table 4.
World reports of Rapidly growing mycobacteria isolated from Central Nervous System after insertion of VP shunt.

and AFB was seen in ZN smear. On culturing on both MGIT and LJ media growth was seen within 7 days. MALDI-TOF identified the isolate as *Mycobacterium fortuitum*. The VP shunt was removed and she was started on Linezolid 10 mg/kg BD, Ofloxacin 20 mg/kg OD, Clofazimine 5 mg/kg OD, Clarithromycin 15 mg/kg BD according to IDSA guidelines on Diagnosis, Treatment and Prevention of Non-tuberculous Mycobacterial Diseases. The patient started improving and her GCS scale improved.

The source of infection in such cases can be nosocomial, trauma, abscess, revision of shunt surgery, and any other surgery performed even after 30 years of VP shunt insertion [53].

NTMs form biofilms on silicone, stainless steel, polyvinyl chloride and polycarbonate of which mostly the present day surgical equipments, catheters and prosthesis comprise of [51, 62]. These come under critical items that enter the sterile space and vascular system. Sterilization of these critical items is recommended by treating with different chemical sterilizing agents but most importantly meticulous cleaning must precede any high-level disinfection or sterilization process.

2.6 Sterilization of medical devices

Spaulding classified the medical instruments as critical, semi-critical and non-critical items (**Table 5**). Non-critical items consists of items which come in contact with patients' intact skin for which surface disinfectants are enough for cleaning. As per critical, semi-critical items which come in contact with sterile spaces and mucous membranes thorough cleaning and disinfection is advised. Though sterilization is the ideal procedure recommended for these items, it is not always possible due to the composition of some of the items e.g. polypropylene. Hence high level disinfection is recommended for these items.

In cases of implants such as VP shunt, venous catheters, orthopedic implants etc. needs to be removed completely. Other than these all critical and semi-critical items are supposed to be treated with high level disinfectants to render it safe for reuse in the next patient (**Table 6**).

Critical items	• Surgical instruments • Cardiac and urinary catheters • Implants • Ultrasound probes
Semi-critical items	• Respiratory therapy and anaesthesia equipment • Endoscopes • Laryngoscope blades • Esophageal manometery probes • Rectal manometery catheters
Non-critical items	• Bedpans • Blood pressure cuffs • Crutches • Bed rails • Bedside tables • Patient furniture

Table 5.
Spaulding classification.

Instruments Used In Hospitals	Sterilization/High Level Disinfection
• Ventriculoperitoneal shunt • Ventriculoarterial shunt • Dental implants	• Removal of implants [63].
• Cardiac /Urinary Catheters • Implants • Ultrsound Probes In Sterile Body Cavities	• Initial manual cleaning with a detergent (soak for 30 min)/enzyme. • Rinse with sterile water. • Blow completely dry with compressed air. • Repackage in sealed envelope. • Sterilize with Ethylene Oxide • Aerate catheters for at least 14 days at room temperature [64, 65].
• Laproscopes • Arthroscopes • Cystoscopes	• Initial manual cleaning with detergent/enzyme. Or • Automated washer/disinfector containing peraccetic acid as liquid disinfectant. • Soak in 2% Glutaraldehyde for 15-20 mins. Or • Orthophthaldehyde (low vapour pressure). Or • Gas plasma technology [66, 67]. • Use of *sterile water* for terminal rinsing.
• G.I. endoscopes • Bronchoscopes • Nasopharyngoscopes	• Clean mechanically internal and external surfaces with detergent/enzymes • Soak in 2% Glutaraldehyde for 15-20 min Or Orthophthaldehyde for 12 min Or 2% Glutaraldehyde @ 25°C ×45 min Or Ethylene Oxide sterilization [68–71]. • Rinse with sterile water. • Dry and rinse the insertion tube and inner channels with alcohol and dry with forced air after disinfection.

Table 6.
Sterilization Procedures for Instruments Used In Hospitals

3. Conclusion

Non-tuberculous mycobacteria may be rare causes of VP shunt-associated infections but should always be considered as a differential diagnosis. However, NTM does not find a mention as an offending organism nor any treatment protocols in the present IDSA guidelines for healthcare-associated ventriculitis and meningitis and management of ventriculo-peritoneal infections in adults. A high index of suspicion based on clinical presentation is essential to diagnose such rare pathogens.

Acknowledgements

I am thankful to Dr Urvashi B. Singh for being a constant support and inspiration for all the members of Tuberculosis laboratory. I am grateful to the technical staff of the laboratory whose tireless efforts have saved patients lives on a daily basis.

Conflict of interest

No conflict of interest.

Author details

Ashit Bhusan Xess*, Kiran Bala and Urvashi B. Singh
All India Institute of Medical Sciences, New Delhi, India

*Address all correspondence to: drurvashi@gmail.com

References

[1] Sáez-Llorens X, McCracken GH. Bacterial meningitis in children. Lancet. 2003;**361**(9375):2139-2148

[2] Kasper DL, Hauser SL, Jameson JL, Fauci AS, Longo DL, Loscalzo J. Harrison'sPrinciplesofInternalMedicine. 19th ed. New York: McGraw Hill Education; 2015

[3] Tunkel AR, Hasbun R, Bhimraj A, Byers K, Kaplan SL, Scheld WM, et al. Infectious Disease Society of America's Clinical Practice guidelines for healthcare-associated ventriculitis and meningitis. Clinical Infectious Diseases. 2017:1-32

[4] Edwards RJ, Drake JM. Cerebrospinal fluid devices. In: Winn HR, editor. Youmans & Winn Neurological Surgery. 7th ed. New York: Elsevier; 2017. pp. 1638-1643

[5] Conen A, Walti LN, Merlo A, Fluckiger U, Battegay M, Trampuz A. Characteristics and treatment outcome of cerebrospinal fluid shunt-associated infections in adults: A retrospective analysis over an 11-year period. Clinical Infectious Diseases. 2008;**47**:73-82

[6] Vinchon M, Dhellemmes P. Cerebrospinal fluid shunt infection: Risk factors and long-term follow-up. Child's Nervous System. 2006;**22**:692-697

[7] van de Beek D, Drake JM, Tunkel AR. Nosocomial bacterial meningitis. The New England Journal of Medicine. 2010;**362**:146-154

[8] Simon TD, Butler J, Whitlock KB, et al. Risk factors for first cerebrospinal fluid shunt infection: Findings from a multi-centre prospective cohort study. Journal of Pediatrics. 2014;**164**:1462-1468 e2

[9] Ramanan M, Lipman J, Shorr A, Shankar A. A meta-analysis of ventriculostomy-associated cerebrospinal fluid infections. BMC Infectious Diseases. 2015;**15**:3

[10] Fjelstad AB, Hommelstad J, Sorteberg A. Infections related to intrathecal baclofen therapy in children and adults: Frequency and risk factors. Journal of Neurosurgery. Pediatrics. 2009;**4**:487-493

[11] Vender JR, Hester S, Waller JL, Rekito A, Lee MR. Identification and management of intrathecal baclofen pump complications: A comparison of pediatric and adult patients. Journal of Neurosurgery. 2006;**104**:9-15

[12] Motta F, Antonello CE. Analysis of complications in 430 consecutive pediatric patients treated with intrathecal baclofen therapy: 14-year experience. Journal of Neurosurgery. Pediatrics. 2014;**13**:301-306

[13] Hester SM, Fisher JF, Lee MR, Macomson S, Vender JR. Evaluation of salvage techniques for infected baclofen pumps in pediatric patients with cerebral palsy. Journal of Neurosurgery. Pediatrics. 2012;**10**:548-554

[14] Stenehjem E, Armstrong WS. Central nervous system device infections. Infectious Disease Clinics of North America. 2012;**26**:89-110

[15] Tsai MH, Lu CH, Huang CR, et al. Bacterial meningitis in young adults in Southern Taiwan: Clinical characteristics and therapeutic outcomes. Infection. 2006;**34**:2-8

[16] Tille PM. Diagnostic Microbiology. 13th ed. St. Louis, Missouri: Elsevier;

[17] Veloci S, Mencarini J, Lagi F, Beltrami G, Campanacci DA, Bartoloni A, et al. Tubercular prosthetic joint infection: Two case reports

and literature review. Infection. 2018;**46**(1):55-68. DOI: 10.1007/s15010-017-1085-1

[18] Barr DA, Whittington AM, White B, Patterson B, Davidson R. Extra-pulmonary tuberculosis developing at sites of previous trauma. The Journal of Infection. 2013;**66**:313-319

[19] Mahale YJ, Aga N. Implant-associated *Mycobacterium tuberculosis* infection following surgical management of fractures: A retrospective observational study. Bone & Joint Journal. 2015;**97-B**:1279-1283

[20] Kadakia AP, Williams R, Langkamer VG. Tuberculous infection in a total knee replacement performed for medial tibial plateau fracture: A case report. Acta Orthopaedica Belgica. 2007;**73**:661-664

[21] Neogi DS, Kumar A, Yadav CS, Singh S. Delayed periprosthetic tuberculosis after total knee replacement: Is conservative treatment possible? Acta Orthopaedica Belgica. 2009;**75**:136-140

[22] Al-Ghamdi B, Widaa HE, Shahid MA, Aladmawi M, Alotaibi J, Sanei AA, et al. Cardiac implantable electronic device infection due to Mycobacterium species: A case report and review of the literature. BMC Research Notes. 2016;**9**(1):414

[23] Tsuyuguchi K, Suzuki K, Sakatani M. Epidemiology of infection by nontuberculous mycobacteria. Respiration and Circulation. 2004;**52**(6):561-564

[24] Falkinham JO III. Surrounded by mycobacteria: Nontuberculous mycobacteria in the human environment. Journal of Applied Microbiology. 2009;**107**(2):356-367

[25] Griffith DE, Aksamit T, Brown-Elliott BA, et al. An official ATS/IDSA statement: Diagnosis, treatment, and prevention of nontuberculous mycobacterial diseases. American Journal of Respiratory and Critical Care Medicine. 2007;**175**(4):367-416

[26] Tortoli E. Clinical manifestations of nontuberculous mycobacteria infections. Clinical Microbiology and Infection. 2009;**15**(10):906-910

[27] Piersimoni C, Scarparo C. Pulmonary infections associated with non-tuberculous mycobacteria in immunocompetent patients. The Lancet Infectious Diseases. 2008;**8**(5):323-334

[28] Horsburgh CR Jr, Gettings J, Alexander LN, Lennox JL. Disseminated *Mycobacterium avium* complex disease among patients infected with human immunodeficiency virus, 1985-2000. Clinical Infectious Diseases. 2001;**33**(11):1938-1943

[29] Esteban J, García-Pedrazuela M, Muñoz-Egea MC, Alcaide F, Current treatment of nontuberculous mycobacteriosis: An update. Expert Opinion on Pharmacotherapy. 2012;**13**(7):967-986

[30] Shamaei M, Marjani M, Farnia P, Tabarsi P, Mansouri D. Human infections due to *Mycobacterium lentiflavum*: First report in Iran. Iranian Journal of Microbiology. 2010;**2**(1):27-29

[31] Al-Anazi KA, Al-Jasser AM, Al-Anazi WK. Infections caused by non-tuberculous mycobacteria in recipients of hematopoietic stem cell transplantation. Frontiers in Oncology. 2014;**4**:article 311, 12 p

[32] El Helou G, Viola GM, Hachem R, Han XY, Raad II. Rapidly growing mycobacterial bloodstream infections. The Lancet Infectious Diseases. 2013;**13**(2):166-174

[33] Löwenstein E. Vorlesungen über Bakteriologie, Immunität, spezifische

Diagnostik und Therapie der Tuberkulose. Jena: Fischer; 1920

[34] Calmette A. L'Infection Bacillaire et la Tuberculose. Paris: Masson et Cie; 1936

[35] Koch R. Classics in infectious diseases. The etiology of tuberculosis: Robert Koch. Berlin, Germany 1882. Reviews of Infectious Diseases. 1982;**4**:1270-1274. DOI: 10.1093/clinids/4.6.1270

[36] Costerton JW, Gessey GC, Cheng KJ. How bacteria stick. Scientific American. 1978;**238**:86-95. DOI: 10.1038/scientificamerican0178-86

[37] Wallace RJ Jr. Nontuberculous mycobacteria and water: A love affair with increasing clinical importance. Infectious Disease Clinics of North America. 1987;**1**:677-686

[38] Schulze-Robbecke R, Fischeder R. Mycobacteria in biofilms. Zentralblatt für Hygiene und Umweltmedizin. 1989;**188**:385-390

[39] Ojha AK, Baughn AD, Sambandan D, Hsu T, Trivelli X, Guerardel Y, et al. Growth of *Mycobacterium tuberculosis* biofilms containing free mycolic acids and harbouring drug-tolerant bacteria. Molecular Microbiology. 2008;**69**:164-174. DOI: 10.1111/j.1365-2958.2008.06274.x

[40] Richards JP, Ojha AK. Mycobacterial biofilms. Microbiology Spectrum. 2014;**2**(5). DOI: 10.1128/microbiolspec.MGM2-0004-2013

[41] Muñoz-Egea MC, García-Pedrazuela M, Mahillo I, García MJ, Esteban J. Autofluorescence as a tool for structural analysis of biofilms formed by nonpigmented rapidly growing mycobacteria. Applied and Environmental Microbiology. 2013;**79**:1065-1067. DOI: 10.1128/AEM.03149-12

[42] Phillips MS, von Reyn CF. Nosocomial infections due to nontuberculous mycobacteria. Clinical Infectious Diseases. 2001;**33**:1363-1374

[43] De Groote MA, Huitt G. Infections due to rapidly growing mycobacteria. Clinical Infectious Diseases. 2006;**42**:1756-1763

[44] Hoefsloot W, van Ingen J, Andrejak C, Angeby K, Bauriaud R, Bemer P, et al. The geographic diversity of nontuberculous mycobacteria isolated from pulmonary samples: A NTM-NET collaborative study. The European Respiratory Journal. 2013;**42**:1604-1613

[45] Carson LA, Petersen NJ, Favero MS, Aguero SM. Growth characteristics of atypical mycobacteria in water and their comparative resistance to disinfectants. Applied and Environmental Microbiology. 1978;**36**:839-846

[46] Le Dantec C, Duguet JP, Montiel A, Dumoutier N, Dubrou S, Vincent V. Chlorine disinfection of atypical mycobacteriaisolated from a water distribution system. Applied and Environmental Microbiology. 2002;**68**:1025-1032

[47] Selvaraju SB, Khan IUH, Yadav JS. Biocidal activity of formaldehyde and nonformaldehyde biocides toward *Mycobacterium immunogenum* and *Pseudomonas fluorescens* in pure and mixed suspensions in synthetic metalworking fluid and saline. Applied and Environmental Microbiology. 2005;**71**:542-546

[48] Bryers JD. Medical biofilms. Biotechnology and Bioengineering. 2008;**100**:1-18

[49] Casadevall A, Pirofski LA. Virulence factors and their mechanisms of action:

The view from a damage-response framework. Journal of Water and Health. 2009;7:S2-S18

[50] Kostakioti M, Hadjifrangiskou M, Hultgren SJ. Bacterial biofilms: Development, dispersal, and therapeutic strategies in the dawn of the post antibiotic era. Cold Spring Harbor Perspectives in Medicine. 2013;**3**:a010306-a010319

[51] Sousa S, Bandeira M, Carvalho PA, Duarte A, Jardao L. Nontuberculous mycobacteria pathogenesis and biofilm assembly. International Journal of Mycobacteriology. 2015;**4**(1):36-43

[52] Talati NJ, Rouphel N, Kuppalli K, Franco-Paredes C. Spectrum of CNS disease caused by rapidly growing mycobacteria. The Lancet Infectious Diseases. 2008;**8**:390-398

[53] Montero JA, Alrabaa SF, Wills TS. *Mycobacterium abscessus* ventriculoperitoneal shunt infection and review of literature. Infection. 2016;**44**:251-253

[54] Baidya A, Tripathi M, Singh UB, Pandey P. *Mycobacterium abscessus* as a cause of chronic meningitis: A rare clinical entity. American Journal of the Medical Sciences. 2016;**351**(4):437-439

[55] Cadena G, Wiedman J, Boggan JE. Ventriculoperitoneal shunt infection with *Mycobacterium fortuitum*: A rare offending organism. Journal of Neurosurgery. Pediatrics. 2014;**14**:704-707

[56] Midani S, Rathore MH. *Mycobacterium fortuitum* infection of ventriculoperitoneal shunt. Southern Medical Journal. 1999;**92**:705-707

[57] Chan KH, Mann KS, Seto WH. Infection of a shunt by *Mycobacterium fortuitum*: Case report. Neurosurgery. 1991;**29**:472-474

[58] Vishwanathan R, Bhagwati SN, Iyer V, Newalkar P. Ventriculo-peritoneal shunt infection by *Mycobacterium fortuitum* in an adult. Neurology India. 2004;**52**:393-394

[59] Alibadi H, Osenbach RK. Intrathecal drug delivery device infection and meningitis due to *Mycobacterium fortuitum*: A case report. Neuromodulation. 2008;**11**:311-314

[60] Madaras-Kelly KJ, Demasters TA, Stevens DL. *Mycobacterium fortuitum* meningitis associated with an epidural catheter: Case report and a review of the literature. Pharmacotherapy. 1999;**19**:661-666

[61] Uche C, Silibovsky R, Jungkind D, Measly R. Ventruloperitoneal shunt associated *Mycobacterium goodie* infection. Infectious Diseases in Clinical Practice. 2008;**16**:129-130

[62] Esteban J, Garcia-Coca M. Mycobacterium biofilms. Frontiers in Microbiology. 2018;**8**:2651. DOI: 10.3389/fmicb.2017.02651. e Collection 2017

[63] Pelegrin I, Lora-Tamayo J, Gomez-Junyent J, Sabe N, Garcia-Somoza D, Gabarros A, et al. Management of ventriculoperitoneal shunt infections in adults. Analysis of risk factors associated with treatment failure. Clinical Infectious Diseases. 2017;**64**(8):989-997

[64] Mayhall CG. Hospital Epidemiology and Infection Control. 3rd ed. Baltimore, Maryland: Lippincott Williams and Wilkins; 2004

[65] Ferrell M, Wolf CE, Ellenbogen KA, Wood MA, Clema HF, Gilligan DM. Ethylene oxide on electrophysiology catheters following resterilization: Implications for catheter reuse. The American Journal of Cardiology. 1997;**80**(12):1558-1561

[66] Rutala WA. 1994, 1995 and 1996 Guideline Committee: APIC guidelines for selection and use of disinfectants. American Journal of Infection Control. 1996;**24**:313-342

[67] Rutala WA, Weber DJ, Committee HICPA Guidelines. Disinfection and sterilization in healthcare facilities: What clinicians need to know. Clinical Infectious Diseases. 2004;**39**(5):702-709

[68] Vesley D, Melson J, Stanley P. Microbial bioburden in endoscope reprocessing and an in-use evaluation of the high level disinfection capabilities of Cidex PA. Gastroenterology Nursing. 1999;**22**(2):63-68

[69] Chu NS, McAlister D, Antonoplos PA. Natural bioburden levels detected on flexible gastrointestinal endoscopes after clinical use and manual cleaning. Gastrointestinal Endoscopy. 1998;**48**(2):137-142

[70] Kruse A, Rey JF. Guidelines on cleaning and disinfection in GI endoscopy. Update 1999. The European Society Of Gastrointestinal Endoscopy. Endoscopy. 2003;**35**:878-881

[71] Hulka JF, Wisler MG, Bruch C. A discussion: Laproscopic instrument sterilization. Medical Instrumentation. 1977;**11**:122-123